The David Levine Affair

Separatist Betrayal or McCarthyism North?

Randal Marlin

Fernwood Publishing • Halifax

To the loving memory of my father
Ervin Ross "Spike" Marlin (1909-1994).

He valued and defended truth.

In deepest appreciation
for so many years of support and guidance.

Editing: Donna Davis
Design and production: Beverley Rach
Printed and bound in Canada by: Hignell Printing Limited

A publication of:
Fernwood Publishing
Box 9409, Station A
Halifax, Nova Scotia
B3K 5S3

Fernwood Publishing Company Limited gratefully acknowledges the financial support
of the Ministry of Canadian Heritage and the Canada Council for the Arts for our
publishing program.

Canadian Cataloguing in Publication Data

Marlin, Randal, 1938—

The David Levine affair

ISBN 1-55266-003-6

1. Levine, David, 1948– -- Public opinion.   2. Ottawa Hospital. Board of Trustees --
Public opinion.   3. Ottawa Hospital -- Administration -- Public opinion.   4. Public
opinion -- Ontario -- Ottawa.   I. Title.

RA983.08209 1998   362.1'1'06071383   C98-950204-X

CONTENTS

Preface and Acknowledgements

The purpose of this book is to record and dissect the elements that went into an extraordinary manifestation of public hysteria in, of all places, Ottawa. It is rare to find an instance where media impact has been so forceful in such a short span of time. David Levine, unknown in the national capital region before May 1, 1998, had by May 19 become known to everyone, an object of heated discussions. One letter writer in *Le Droit* compared the furore over Levine's appointment as CEO of the newly amalgamated Ottawa Hospital to the uproar in Paris almost exactly a hundred years ago when French opinion was divided over Captain Alfred Dreyfus.

There are obvious differences in these cases, but the hatreds and fears evoked were similar. A form of nationalist or patriotic pride was at the centre of both. And in both cases dispassionate concern for refined truth gave way to flag-waving insistence on an overriding verity—the nation. When Emile Zola published his celebrated defence of Dreyfus on January 13, 1898, people called him a traitor and a Prussian spy. In both cases, concerns for truth or civil liberties got steamrolled under the crowd's paramount concern for the integrity (moral in one case, territorial in the other) of the nation. Once a mob is excited and has a rallying focal point, raising sceptical doubts has no impact. The sceptic is simply lumped in with the enemy.

In Ottawa the enemy was separatism, and Levine became targeted as a symbol of separatism. Therefore anyone who spoke in defence of his freedom of opinion became an enemy, part of what William Weintraub calls the "Lamb Lobby." In Act II Scene 2 of his 1998 satirical play *The Underdogs,* Weintraub describes the Lamb Lobby as "a group of philosophers ... who told us that if we cringed enough and grovelled enough we wouldn't get kicked. They called it 'building bridges.'" Although the mob in Ottawa did not use that particular expression, it represents what many of them had in mind. Those federalists who spoke out at the May 19 meeting in favour of Levine's right to freedom of opinion ran a strong risk of being labelled a separatist.

The crowd gathered at the May 19 press conference was quite certain of itself—David Levine incarnated separatism and he had to go, along with the Ottawa Hospital board that hired him. One might think that a Jewish anglophone, who learned French at age 25, would hardly be inclined to promote separatism, especially in Ontario. But enough had been said and repeated in the media to make the crowd secure in its belief that Levine would be promoting separatist fortunes if his appointment were not rescinded.

In Canada, separatism, the movement for Quebec secession or sovereignty as some call it, is promoted by two legitimately elected parties, the Parti Québécois and the Bloc Québécois. Close to half the Quebec population believes, at least from time to time, in that option. Although some may feel that this option should not be allowed, Canadians have not outlawed it and the Supreme Court of Canada decided on August 20, 1998, that secession would be legitimate if certain conditions were met. How could it be, then, that the crowd gathered in Ottawa would be so ready to label as "traitor" a person who once supported what is after all a legitimate political party?

One important factor was the media's handling of the issue. People take their behavioural cues from others, particularly when the others in question are known to be simultaneously reaching tens or hundreds of thousands of people in their area. Attitudes get formed, and when a majority of like-minded people gather to vent some powerful emotions, they often experience a giddy sense of empowerment. An emotional crowd can be very dangerous. Although the experience of the Levine affair was short-lived, it is very instructive and can serve as a warning against fanning the flames of controversy where sensitive issues are involved and where careful attention to fact and detail are needed.

This book documents the progression of the media coverage of David Levine's CEO appointment in various stages: the initial announcement on May 1 and extensive publicity given to opponents of the appointment; the May 15 press conference, with even more hostile reaction when Levine declined to renounce his separatist past; the May 19 meeting, coverage of that meeting and reaction to it; and finally, the aftermath, which has not yet been entirely played out. As recently as September 2, 1998, the *Ottawa Citizen* reported that Quebec deputy premier Bernard Landry said he was "proud" to count David Levine among his separtist party's supporters, prompting a brief renewal of the controversy.

Unfortunate time constraints have required a hasty treatment, but I hope that readers will get a sense of how the impact of the media is cumulative, and how repetition of facts and rumours creates a sense of certainty when this may not be warranted. The overall merits of the different cases to be made for or against separatism, the wisdom of the original hiring, the relative treatments of linguistic minorities in Quebec and Ontario, and so on, are beyond the scope of this book.

I happen to believe that David Levine was a good choice for chief executive officer of the Ottawa Hospital, but the information provided by the board on June 9 should have been presented much earlier. There are obvious limits to the principle that a person's private beliefs and commitments have no bearing on his or her fitness for public office, but it is not within the scope of this book to argue the exact extent of those limits. As will become apparent, however, I believe the case for rescinding the Levine appointment was inadequate, and that doing so would have been calamitous. Readers can make up their own minds on these matters. I hope to encourage sober reconsideration of whatever beliefs people may have formed at the time. Newspapers are read, radio stations are listened to, and the messages are absorbed without people knowing exactly where they got their ideas, whether from a reliable source or from a misleading headline or talk-show rumours. With this in mind, I have tried to provide accurate documentation for what transpired in Ottawa—a media test-tube situation that provides an ideal subject for analysis.

I owe thanks to many people and institutions. Carleton University's MacOdrum library and St. Pat's Resource Centre, the National Library of Canada, the Parliamentary Library, and the Ottawa City Public Library gave me access to all necessary newspapers. The *Ottawa Citizen, Ottawa Sun, Le Droit, Le Devoir* and many individuals gave me permission to reprint materials, for which I am grateful. Thanks to Janet Carson, Susan Jackson and Nancy Peden at the MacOdrum Library and Barbara Harris at St. Pat's. Thanks also to the many interviewees whose names appear in the text. Different people were helpful in different ways; some were very encouraging, while others provided forceful challenges to some of my initial assumptions, leading me to revise my thinking or re-articulate my ideas. Among Carleton friends and colleagues I would especially like to thank André Elbaz, Bob Gould, Henry Mayo, Don McEown, Blair Neatby, Sinclair Robinson, Conrad Winn and Marion Dewar. I appreciate also the responsiveness of Nick Mulder, Sol Shinder, Judy Brown, Brad Mann, Maria Bohuslawsky, Scott Anderson, Brian Sarjeant, Garry Guzzo, William Johnson, Reuel Amdur, Dale Hibbard, Clive Doucet, Alex Munter, Peter Clark, Rabbi Reuben Bulka, Denis Pitt and Charles Shaver. Thanks to George Potter, Stuart Busat, Ray Dean, Dick Flint, Iona Skuce and Marguerite Ritchie for helping me to better understand some of the anti-Levine concerns, and to Hubert Gratton for spelling out his pro-francophone, anti-separatist, pro-Levine position with useful references and observations. I am grateful to Gerry Cammy of CFRA Radio and Wade Wallace and Frank Laverty for a worthwhile on-air exchange. I had the benefit of discussions with colleagues on the Civil Liberties Association—National Capital Region—and with contributors to the Propaganda and Media bulletin board of National Capital Freenet. Special thanks to Conrad Winn of COMPAS Research for providing material from the *Ottawa Citizen*-sponsored public opinion survey, included in the Appendix.

Without the initial encouragement of Fernwood publisher Errol Sharpe it is unlikely that this project would have taken flight. He also gave important advice about how to structure this book and some useful corrections. Many thanks to Donna Davis for numerous stylistic improvements. I would above all like to thank my daughter Christine and my wife Elaine, both of whom read the whole text and made many helpful suggestions. The list could go on at length, but I want to assure everyone with whom I have spoken on the matter that I am grateful for their assistance.

The future of Canada is difficult to predict. My greatest hope for this book is that it will discourage vindictive attitudes and promote an atmosphere in which civilized discourse and respect for individuals with whom one may disagree profoundly, will take precedence over cherished political ideals. There are three forerunners for this kind of thinking: Albert Camus, George Orwell and Jacques Ellul, the last of whom warned us against "the political illusion," the idea that somehow life's major problems can be solved by getting the right people elected, or the right constitution, or the right political formula. These are all important, but none of them will work without the right spirit, including tolerance, among those whom the political system is meant to serve. Camus, echoing St. Augustine, warned that enthusiastic seekers for an otherwise worthy goal discredit that goal when they use illicit means to achieve it.

It would be contrary to the spirit of this main objective to harp on imperfections in the mass media. They have a difficult task to perform with many difficult value judgements to make every day and very little time in which to make them. Mistakes were made. There was in fact some demagoguery, maybe even some unworthy motivation. But I have no desire to encourage a media hate campaign. If what appears here encourages those in the media to think a little more about social responsibility, and consumers of the media to view what they read and hear more critically, then I shall be very satisfied. If it can also stimulate earnest and respectful reflection about minority rights, freedom of belief and expression, and the need to accommodate Quebec's special concerns—hopefully within a continuing Canada—so much the better.

Introduction

On the evening of May 19, 1998, an ugly, noisy, militant and uncompromising face of English Canada was presented to the world. An overflow crowd had gathered in an Ottawa auditorium to confront the board of the newly amalgamated Ottawa Hospital over the choice of David Levine as the new top administrator. The crowd sought the resignation of Levine and the board. Chants of "Out! out! out!" "Resign!" "Mulder [Nick Mulder, chair of the board] must go!" "The board's got to go!" peppered the meeting.

The objection? David Levine was a separatist. He had run for the Parti Québécois in 1979, and was currently serving as a Quebec government envoy in New York. Public opposition was being reported in the media and the board was there to listen. Some distinguished defenders of the Levine appointment, such as former mayor Marion Dewar, were booed and shouted down. "O Canada" was sung several times, inside and outside the auditorium.

How and why, in a generally civilized city and country, did this happen? Canadians have been accustomed to regarding McCarthyism as a phenomenon south of the border. Yet here was one of the same basic ingredients: a strident patriotism, which reduced complex questions to a simple us-and-them mentality. To be for Levine, in this simplistic thinking, was to be for separatism and against Canada. To be soft on separatism, the "break-up" of Canada, was to be un-Canadian. The animosity extended to opponents of the mob mentality, so that those who spoke out in favour of free speech also courted the charge of "separatist."

Prior to the May 19 meeting, letters to newspaper editors and calls to radio talk shows poured out in quantities unparalleled in recent memory[1] and seized public attention. Both of Ottawa's major newspapers called for Mr. Levine's resignation, despite the generally accepted and well-buttressed claim that, political concerns aside, he was by far the most capable person, among the applicants, to handle this demanding job.

What started out as a local concern quickly reached the provincial and then federal levels. Prime Minister Jean Chrétien, Intergovernmental Affairs Minister Stéphane Dion, Ontario Premier Michael Harris, Quebec Premier Lucien Bouchard and Quebec Liberal leader Jean Charest all spoke out on the issue. On May 21 the Quebec legislature passed a motion defending Levine and condemning intolerance. Questions were asked in the House of Commons. Columns and editorials were written from Vancouver to Halifax. The subject was debated on CBC's Cross-Country Checkup. Politicians were called upon to take sides—either calling for tolerance or supporting the anti-Levine forces, which to appearances were in the majority and possessed of more deeply held feelings.

George Orwell knew well the power of a mob. He felt it as a police officer in Burma when, against his better judgement, he caved in to the pressure of an angry crowd and shot a blameless elephant. He also knew the power of a stereotyped, nationalistic view of the world. He knew how ordinary human decency and respect for another person can be overshadowed by party feeling, group belonging and flag waving.[2]

The group gathered at the Civic site of the Ottawa Hospital on May 19 was emotional and excited to an unhealthy degree—in short, hysterical—and not what one would call a representative sample of the population of Ottawa. Many came in answer to appeals from the anti-Levine media or from friends in various organized groups. Most were of retirement age or close to it. No bullets were fired. The assaults were verbal. But disrespect and unreason were rampant. The dominant philosophy was that Canada is one country, a great country for which men and women had made great sacrifices, had even died. This country is indivisible and attempts to break it up are treasonous. Furthermore, anyone who believes that Canada may be broken up is shameful, and anyone who has actively worked toward that end should be made to suffer— they should certainly not be rewarded with a plum $330,000 job.

That was the steamroller set of beliefs, reinforced by medal-wearing, World War II veterans who could challenge most of those who spoke differently on an *ad hominem* basis. "I was willing to die for my country. What have you done to justify your belief?" was the undercurrent of support for their credibility.

It is useless, under such circumstances, to appeal to pragmatic considerations or to softer abstractions, such as the Canadian Charter of Rights and Freedoms, which guarantees freedom of opinion and association. Useless, that is, to argue that maybe showing tolerance towards a separatist might send some favourable signal to Quebec: "Hey, we understand why you people have wanted to leave Canada. You don't feel at home here. Well, look. We recognize your desire to be different, and we'll welcome you among us. We hope that in this welcoming you'll see that you don't need to separate but can thrive in this great country, Canada." This book is a forum for the kinds of things that could not be said at that meeting and can now be aired. We are dealing not just with a local issue, but with a problem that is at the core of the Canadian unity debate. The Levine affair is a microcosm of suspicion, mistrust and misunderstanding that could someday be repeated on a larger scale with worse consequences.

The media, with their own agenda, played an important role in fanning the flames of this controversy. When the news first broke about the hiring of David Levine, the media emphasized not his unusual competence as an administrator, but his close ties with the Parti Québécois in Quebec, including his candidacy for the party in 1979. Nor was there adequate consideration of the motives he might have had for supporting that party, in particular its socially progressive policies at that time or his desire to assist Quebec's fortunes without seeking especially to promote separation from Canada. From the beginning, media treatment heightened awareness of characteristics that would fuel opposition to the appointment and contribute to divisiveness rather than accommodation in the community.

The framework for the perception of Levine's appointment was laid down by the *Citizen*, which published the news on May 1, ahead of all other media. The story was picked up by radio, in particular CFRA's Lowell Green, who revisited the issue many times in the following weeks to accommodate an unprecedented audience response. The *Citizen* also kept the issue alive with stories, letters, commentary and editorials. The emphasis on Levine's particularly suitable capabilities was slow in coming. The issue of human rights, of freedom of belief and association, was also slow to be addressed, coming to the fore in the *Citizen* May 17, though mentioned in an article May 15 on Bloc Québécois Leader Gilles Duceppe, and aired on CBC television. By that time public impressions had become fixed. Separatism was the issue, not freedom of opinion.

The two Ottawa-based English-language daily newspapers were of the same mind: the Levine hiring was a mistake; he should resign or the board should dismiss him. Considerable exposure was given to the views of MPP Garry Guzzo, who was first quoted as saying, "I'd want the board to be satisfied that his loyalties lie with Canada ...," and later, in the May 8 *Ottawa Citizen*, that Levine would be likely to fill "the whole administration with separatists" as he "begins to hire his own staff."

In such an environment, the uproar that characterized the meeting of May 19 was hardly surprising. CFRA listeners and *Ottawa Sun* readers were encouraged to get to the meeting early and be heard: be at the meeting, denounce the Levine appointment and thereby save Canada.

Not all the media were anti-Levine; the *Globe and Mail* and the CBC, for example, were not. But the influence of the *Globe* came only mid-way in the month, with the first story, by Graham Fraser, on May 14. Fraser focused on Levine's superb credentials and on the oddity of the capital region reacting "as though Mr. Levine had been recruited from a terrorist organization."

Not surprisingly, the French-language press had a very different perspective on David Levine. For Franco-Ontarians in the area, concerned that they not lose out on services in their own language with the shifting role of the Montfort Hospital, Levine's commitment to the principle of bilingual services was welcome. In Montreal the separatist-leaning newspapers saw the issue as one of freedom of belief. To fire Levine on the basis of his separatist convictions would be to violate the Canadian Charter of Rights and Freedoms, they argued, and in any event would belie federalist boasts about Canada being the world's most tolerant democracy.

There was thus a deep rift in perception of the David Levine affair by French and English language media. While the *Citizen* eventually presented the case for Levine's right to freedom of opinion, the three French papers tracked in my study (*Le Devoir, Le Journal de Montréal,* and *Le Droit*) typically shunned a sympathetic treatment of the "traitor" viewpoint. In their view responsible people were to denounce such nonsense and political leaders were called to account for signs of hesitancy, ambiguity or tergiversation on the point.[3]

The aim of this book is to analyse the "Levine affair," focusing on the media that tended to incite the crowd—at first the *Ottawa Citizen* and CFRA Radio, and then the *Ottawa Sun*—the affair is not adequately represented simply as a straightforward conflict between diehard federalists and separatists, nor as a conflict between anglophones and francophones, nor even as a conflict between civil libertarians and united Canada patriots. Each of those conflicts is present, but there is much more. There is, for example, the frustration caused by a sense of powerlessness. Linda McQuaig has described this phenomenon in her book with the pertinent title, *The Culture of Impotence.* Many technological changes are happening, and too often the ordinary citizen has little say in them. The Levine hiring was once more an unelected board making decisions that directly affected people's lives. The board itself was not presented with a shortlist by the selection committee but was asked to approve the committee's choice. Not only that, but a headline announcing the appointment appeared in the *Ottawa Citizen* on the same morning, May 1, that the board was scheduled to approve it. Management of the PR aspects of the appointment was clearly at fault and did not contribute to public confidence in the board or its choice.

Also in the background, though perhaps at a deeper level, is a sense of frustration among many people that has been brought about by the loss of symbols of Canadian unity. Social programs and the safety net constructed following the Second World War signified a Canada people could take pride in. Education was extended, loans were provided so that students lacking financial means could still get a university education. Medical care was to be available to rich and poor alike. People who fought for their country could look forward to a decent life for their children.

This was a Canada worthy of sacrifices. When Pierre Trudeau became prime minister in 1968 and began to promote bilingualism in the civil service, many unilingual English civil servants learned French. Those who didn't, and even some who did, found their careers held back. In the name of Canadian unity, it still seemed worthwhile though. Then came additional demands from Quebec, the "two nations" theory and Brian Mulroney in 1984 taking further steps to accommodate Quebec's demands, opening up high positions in his government to known separatists. When Lucien Bouchard then set up his own federal separatist party it seemed a betrayal to some, though of course from another perspective it could be seen simply as a logical step towards achieving certain French aspirations. Panic over the deficit in the 1980s led to reductions in federal transfer payments and a decline in commitment to social programs. Education, health care and funding for cultural institutions have suffered huge cuts. Family allowances disappeared for the middle class. Pensions are uncertain in a world of increasing clawbacks. Having stomached separatists in the federal government, reached retirement age, and set their sights on medical care for themselves and a good education for their children, many anglophone retired civil servants or military personnel were suddenly faced with what seemed to them a huge insult—another separatist, this time in an Ontario-funded institution. The intolerable thought occurred to them that employment in the Ontario public service, jobs paid for by Ontario taxpayers, might be withheld from their unilingual anglophone children or grandchildren. The spectre of being cared for, perhaps even dying, in a hospital where the staff speak French to each other was disheartening to some.[4]

Those who do not feel this way are sometimes sympathetic to the feelings of those who do, acknowledging that the way in which the Levine appointment was arrived at and presented to the public was tactless to say the least.

H. Blair Neatby, Professor Emeritus of History at Carleton University in Ottawa, has suggested some additional reasons why the reaction against the Levine appointment should be so emotional and deep-rooted.

> The explanation, I think, requires some analysis of the social context in Ottawa and the restructuring of the Ottawa hospitals. The Ottawa General was founded by an Order of French-speaking, Roman Catholic nuns. It is now some 20 years or so since the General became a non-sectarian institution, but to many in Ottawa the General is still thought of as Roman Catholic. And because it is "bilingual" (meaning it provides services in both English and French) it is seen by many as predominantly French. The Civic, on the other hand, has always been non-denominational but is thought of by many as Protestant. The Civic also offers some services in French, but many think of it as the English-language hospital.
>
> Hospital restructuring in Ottawa was therefore a minefield of religious and linguistic fears. The mass rally for the Montfort Hospital illustrates the intensity of the fears of the minority that French services would be curtailed. [On March 22, 1997, some 10,000 flag-waving, anthem-singing Franco-Ontarians gathered at Ottawa's Civic Centre to protest the threatened closure of the French-language Ottawa hospital. The rally, greatly supported by *Le Droit*, which published an unusual special edition, led to a decision in August that year to keep the hospital open, but with a reduced function.]

> The merger of the General and the Civic was the flashpoint for various groups of English-speaking citizens who saw the Civic as "their" hospital. They could interpret the merger as subordinating the Civic to the General. There are some valid grounds for this interpretation—the General has newer buildings and is located at the centre of a health-services complex. And it is also true that the merger will be very disruptive—the identity of both hospitals has been based to a significant degree on institutional rivalry and the merger will certainly involve major adjustments in the institutional cultures. So it is not unreasonable to believe that the Civic, as people have known it, is facing major changes.[5]

The fear arising from these changes was that the Civic would be forced to become "bilingual," with the anticipated result that hospital staff would have to learn French and that unilingual doctors and nurses would lose their jobs, perhaps to French-speaking appointees from Quebec.[6] Hearing how language laws are applied in Quebec adds to the tension. Reports that an experienced doctor was leaving the Montreal Children's Hospital for a position in the United States because he failed a French language test, and that unilingual French signs were imposed in what was once a hospital for the English-speaking population (Brome-Missisquoi-Perkins), created apprehension in some minds for what might come to Ottawa.[7]

That David Levine should be the object of this hostility may seem surprising. English was his mother-tongue; it was not until he was in his mid-twenties that he learned French. Being Jewish, he is not on one side or other of the Catholic-Protestant divide. The job as top administrator of the Ottawa Hospital demands a knowledge about how to restructure services effectively and the diplomatic skills to get the changes accepted—skills that he clearly possesses. How then did he become the target of so much animosity? Professor Neatby adds his theory to the others:

> Fears have little respect for facts. Levine became the scapegoat or the lightning rod. If he hadn't had PQ connections it would have been necessary to find some other aspect of his identity to attack. He is bilingual—but any successful candidate had to be bilingual. To the critics, however, being bilingual means that he is pro-French (that is, it means that he is the threat or the enemy). His separatist connections become the irrefutable proof that he is one of "them" and not one of "us." It thus becomes obvious that Levine will make the Civic a French (and maybe more Catholic?) institution if he is allowed to.
>
> There is a logic to this—but it is a logic which can only appeal to those who feel that their place in society is threatened and their institutions are under attack. The Levine incident is revealing because it

shows that some citizens feel that their status has been threatened by the changes in Ottawa over the last thirty years. If Levine hadn't existed he would have had to be invented. Or, more accurately, the Levine of the *Citizen* and the *Sun* and of the placards ....

What remains to be seen is how powerful the hostile forces are and whether Levine will find enough support in the community for the very difficult decisions he will have to make.[8]

The pressure on the hospital board to rescind Levine's appointment was immense. As mentioned, both the *Ottawa Citizen* and the *Ottawa Sun* called for his resignation, and many letters denouncing the appointment were published. Premier Mike Harris and Health Minister Elizabeth Witmer made public statements suggesting that maybe the board should rethink its position.

Despite the pressure, the board refused to cave in and reaffirmed Levine's appointment. Many federalists heaved a sigh of relief. The French media were treating the event as a test-case for anglo good faith. Already, separatists had been able to exploit the situation for their own ends. Once the appointment was upheld, though, the incident became of less concern to the Montreal French-language media.

Seldom does a body of such heated opinion get formed so quickly. David Levine went from being an unknown entity to a name recognized by most of the adult population in Ottawa. Even people across Canada recognize the name and the issue.[9] In tracking the build up of opinion, which culminated in the uproarious, venomous meeting of May 19, I have systematically studied every May issue of the *Ottawa Sun*, the *Ottawa Citizen*, the *Globe and Mail, Le Journal de Montréal, Le Devoir* and *Le Droit*. I have also interviewed letter writers, politicians and people who have interesting views on the subject. I have also purchased the two most important tapes of the Lowell Green talk-in radio program heard on CFRA Radio, and have studied the CPAC complete broadcast of the May 19 meeting. I would have liked to extend the scope of this study to include CBC TV and CJOH as well as other electronic media and newspapers, but time constraints made this impossible.

The response of the French-language media merits study. From their perspective, the hostility to Levine represented intolerance of what has for over twenty years been treated as a legitimate democratic option—that of separating from the rest of Canada should Quebecers so choose. The display of hostility re-created the kind of feeling that occurred with the rejection of the Meech Lake agreement, which leads to increased support for Quebec sovereignty. The existence of this feeling provides the basis for a pragmatic assessment that a strong anti-separatist measure of dubious legality, such as rescinding Mr. Levine's appointment, would be counterproductive, actually increasing the chances of separation.

Although the media had an important role in what transpired, it would be ridiculous to think that the highly emotional response to Levine was of their own creation. There was incitement, but there was also a set of pre-existing attitudes that were surprisingly receptive to such incitement. The following chapters examine the ways in which the media used a catalogue of old and new fears, suspicions and resentments to create, fan and exploit controversy. The *Ottawa Citizen*'s new editor is implementing a deliberate policy to create controversy, to be talked about, to increase circulation. Under this policy, it is important not to confuse people by hitting them with two or more conflicting ideas on the same day. The aim is to present one side of the conflict one day, or over the course of a few days, and then present the other side. It seems to work, in that it generates lots of letters, sometimes very thoughtful ones. But the effect of presenting only one side of a highly charged, emotional issue can be socially disruptive, as the Levine affair shows.

Some good may result, but there are those who believe the Levine affair courted serious damage to the fabric of this country. Ottawa-Carleton Regional Councillor Clive Doucet was of the opinion that if the hospital board had yielded to public pressure and fired Levine, Premier Bouchard would have had just what he needed to sway public opinion in Quebec to win the next referendum.[10] The new head of Alliance Quebec, William Johnson, did not see it as quite so influential, but he thought it would certainly give Bouchard important ammunition.[11] A poll by the Léger & Léger polling firm in Quebec concluded that the Levine controversy "reinforced the negative views of many Quebecers about the attitudes of English-speaking Canadians."[12]

With respect to the factors affecting the emotional response to the Levine choice, some additional points are worth adding. The English-speaking population in Ottawa includes a fair number of people who came from Quebec following the October 1970 crisis, which itself had been preceded by Westmount mail-bombings and other acts of intimidation. Language laws, such as Bill 101, gave an additional signal that the workplace was to be in French, and those unwilling to learn the language were often told that for advancement they should leave the province.

To the resentments already described, there is the already mentioned Canada-wide alarm at the erosion of the health care system. One cause is the reduction in federal transfer payments to the provinces. But there is also a neo-conservative or neo-liberal philosophy which sees the old safety net as removing incentives and self-reliance, which is also a convenient excuse for introducing private care to replace the public system and generate profits. Some suspect that the degeneration of the health care system is part of a conspiracy to increase the demand for private health care services in Canada. This would be consistent with a generalized selfishness among the rich, who perhaps want to see fewer dollars supporting the general population and more dollars supporting their own interests. This approach has an impact on "high-tech" medicine, since some of it is too costly for the average Canadian. It would be con-

venient for the wealthy if apportionment were decided on the basis of fee payments instead of some objective, health-determined reason more in keeping
with the spirit of the Canada Health Act.

High-tech developments have also produced the potential for huge sav-
ings, however. Dr. Wilburt Keon, noted Ottawa heart specialist, has pointed
out that people who were formerly confined to hospital beds are now able to
live in their homes with appropriate heart-monitoring devices. But not everyone can go home to an adequate health support system. The care needed may
be minimal, but without it getting the right dosage of medicine at the right time
or an adequate diet becomes a matter of life and death. Some elderly people
need assistance to move around the house, get out of bed and go to the bath-
room. As hospitals close, more and more infirm people need these home-care
services, and there are horror stories about this help not being forthcoming. We
put all factors together, we are faced with a roiling pot of multiple fears and
resentments: health care and the principle of universal accessibility, hospital
treatment in congenial surroundings, the future of Canada, jobs, bilingualism,
responsiveness from government, and so on.

There may also be an element of class resentment involved in the Levine
case, fuelled by the large salary that went with the position. The figure of
$330,000 a year is not out of line for someone who heads the third largest
hospital in Canada, but it is far beyond the reach of the average Canadian and
will no doubt seem excessive in the light of hefty cutbacks in medical care
spending. There is resentment against the educated elite who seem not to care
much about the opinions of the masses, and the latter feel they are dismissed as
a rabble not to be taken seriously. It is always dangerous for an elite to give the
impression of showing contempt for those who do not share in their privileges.
For this and similar reasons, some have suggested that hospital boards be either directly elected or accountable to a committee of an elected body, such as
the Regional Council of Ottawa-Carleton.[13]

Against the background described, it is easy to see that acceptance of David
Levine as head of the Ottawa Hospital would require a great deal of trust. His
separatist background made this difficult despite his good-faith promises. For
example, Levine explicitly denied that he would show favouritism or demand
that all hospital staff be bilingual. Some people felt however, that, as a separatist, he had betrayed his own anglophone community in Montreal and lacked
trustworthiness generally. Such a viewpoint smacks of prejudice. It was clear
that Levine was mainly concerned with the socially progressive policies of the
PQ at the time. It is not necessarily a betrayal, and on the face of things quite
the opposite, to attempt to "build bridges" with the anglophone community.

It was also held against Levine that he would not divulge his current political beliefs regarding separatism. Lowell Green, of CFRA Radio, has noted
on air that Levine, when specifically asked whether he had pledged an oath of
allegiance to the separatist cause, replied first with "No" and then qualified his

answer by referring to his earlier hospital appointment in Montreal rather than to his more recent appointment as Quebec envoy to New York. Levine seemed to take the position that his political beliefs should only be divulged when relevant to the job he will perform. He clearly believed that these were not of special relevance in his new posting. It is a principled position, though pragmatically precarious.

Another specific grievance fuelling passions in Ottawa was and is resentment against Quebecers for using Ottawa hospitals and not paying the full costs. Dr. Charles Shaver has brought this point to public attention with numerous letters and articles in newspapers and other publications. The Quebec government has shown a reluctance to pay the full cost of the Ontario fees when Quebec patients are treated there, even though this is contrary to the Canada Health Act. A special agreement has been negotiated to remove this irritant, but because many loopholes remain, doctors or hospitals are often left short-changed. Added to this is another well-publicized grievance that Ontario construction workers have work barred from them in Quebec, but that the converse is not true.

Of course, David Levine has nothing to do with these particular grievances, which existed before he was even considered a candidate for heading the Ottawa Hospital. But a certain proportion of the people, as shown by the crowd assembled to jeer the board that selected him, clearly feared that he would do much to benefit Quebec, and not so much to benefit the anglo population of this corner of Ontario. Once again, we deal with prejudicial judgements.

In Chapter One I will recount, chronologically, the media treatment of the Levine affair prior to the May 15 press conference. I will note what took place in the different media, but will reserve my overall systematic analysis and evaluation for Chapter Five. I will underscore the different perspectives in both French and English media. This is one issue where Conrad Black cannot be accused of imposing uniformity in the media he controls: the stance taken by *Le Droit* and the *Ottawa Citizen*, both of them Ottawa dailies under Black's Hollinger, Inc. media empire, was very different.

In Chapter Two I examine the period from the day of the press conference May 15 until the meeting of May 19. Chapter Three deals with the meeting itself and the reaction to it, the period of nation-wide attention. Chapter Four picks up the story after the Ottawa board stood firm on its commitment to hire Levine, and announced its stand May 21. In Chapter Five I analyse some of the key problems in the Levine affair and arrive at some conclusions. I have included notes based on interviews with various letter writers. The interviews were carried out partly to see how strongly a writer felt and whether other considerations might lead them to revise their opinion. I spoke with people who were actively involved in the community, who possessed special knowledge or who were involved in some special way in the unfolding saga. I spoke with board members and anti-Levine agitators, including MPP Garry Guzzo.

The David Levine affair gave us in miniature a preview of the kind of passionate awakening that can easily be a prelude to violence. It showed that for a brief period reason took second place to emotion. The media at times presented a one-sided picture—which side depended for a while on which language was spoken on air or printed in the newspaper one read.

It often happens with what we learn through the media that the sources of beliefs and prejudices are eventually forgotten, leaving only the impressions. By publishing a record of events, I hope to do several things. First, I want to increase public perception about how beliefs might have been formed, so that people will become more cautious about how the media might sway them. Second, I would like to keep attention focused on the issues that caused the disturbance. The media are preoccupied with the issues of the moment and move on. I wish to encourage greater self-examination in our society about issues connected with the Levine affair. Third, evidence in this book supports a curb on the media policy of exciting maximum controversy in society. Fear-mongering, and treating other legitimate groups with contempt must be avoided if peace is to be maintained. I advocate self-restraint and the pressure of public opinion, not any law. I hope that those who disagree with my analysis will put forward their own different opinions in a spirit of enlightenment rather than of polemic, since respectful disagreement is part of what this book is all about.

NOTES

1. This statement is made on the basis of interviews with Ronnie Roberts, producer of the Lowell Green radio phone-in program on CFRA Radio, Ottawa, and with Brian Sarjeant, letters editor of the *Ottawa Citizen,* neither of whom could remember any other topic which aroused as much interest or emotion.

2. See the essays, "Notes on Nationalism," and "Shooting an Elephant," in George Orwell, Collected Essays, London: Mercury Books, 1961.

3. For the sake of balance it may be worth recalling that after the vote was taken on patriation of the Canadian Constitution, including the Charter of Rights, a full-page advertisement by La société Saint-Jean-Baptiste de Montréal appeared in *Le Devoir* on December 4, headed "Ce sont des traîtres" ("These people are traitors") with names of the Quebec MPs who had voted in favour. This was followed the next day by an apology from Jean-Louis Roy, the newspaper's publisher, saying that the advertisement had not been vetted by the top management, and that publication would have been refused if it had been. See also the *Globe and Mail,* February 3, 1982, "Court rules 'traitors' posters are fair political comment."

4. I want to thank former Ottawa Mayor Marion Dewar for suggesting points about insecurity resulting from erosion of the commitment to social programs. I also want to share concerns, among both French and English, about the need for treatment in a hospital which is language-friendly to the patient. Mr. Levine appears to have been prejudicially regarded as insensitive on this issue, when he has himself expressed sensitivity to the problem. Sometimes the PQ, with which he was associated, gives cause for concern, most recently when officials of the Office de la

Langue Française decided that two of three nurses at Montreal's Chinese hospital would not need to speak a Chinese language, even though they reportedly would be looking after elderly patients who speak neither English nor French. (See William Johnson, "An offence to decency," *Ottawa Sun*, July 31, 1998.)

5. H. Blair Neatby, personal communication included with permission, June 18, 1998.

6. See Neatby, *supra* note 5.

7. See Keith Henderson, leader of Quebec's Equality Party, "Doctors and nurses subject to strictures of language laws," *Financial Post*, May 6, 1998.

8. See Neatby, *supra* note 5.

9. Reasons for this interest are in Barbara Yaffe's column, "Why David Levine is more than an Ottawa story," in the *Vancouver Sun*, May 22, 1998.

10. Clive Doucet, interview, week of June 1, 1998.

11. William Johnson, interview, week of June 1, 1998.

12. Richard Mackie, "Charest's lead holds up, poll finds," *Globe and Mail*, May 30, 1998, p. 1. The poll was conducted between May 21 and 27 "when the attacks on Mr. Levine's appointment reached their peak," according to the story. I would dispute this claim. The attacks on Levine reached their peak in the combined Ottawa media around May 15 and 16. The public made its fiercest protest at the meeting on May 19. The *Ottawa Sun*'s attacks continued through that week, but the *Citizen* as a whole had become more Levine-friendly. Reports on the Levine protest reached their peak in the Quebec media in the few days following the May 19 meeting. But once the board stood by its decision, on May 21, the basis for some of the Quebec indignation was taken away, though the momentum generated by reports on the May 19 meeting led to extensive coverage until May 23 and beyond.

13. See, for example, Regional Councillor Alex Munter's argument, "Why hospital boards should go," *Ottawa Citizen*, May 20, C4. He and Councillor Madeleine Meilleur have co-authored a discussion paper, "Keeping Ottawa-Carleton Healthy," June 1998, which focuses on the need for an official who is charged with overseeing the effectiveness of the whole health delivery system at the regional level and with responding to public concerns.

CHAPTER ONE

THE ANNOUNCEMENT AND FIRST PRESS CONFERENCE, MAY 1

The angry, flag-waving, "O Canada" singing crowd that confronted the hospital board in the Civic site amphitheatre on May 19 was not simply manufactured, but neither did it just happen spontaneously. A slant in media coverage encouraged a negative view of the appointment of David Levine as CEO of the Ottawa Hospital. As time went on, editorials, columnists and letters called for Levine's resignation. The strongly condemnatory word "treason" was allowed to appear in letters, with seemingly no restraining or critical voice from the editorial corner. As a result, the ugly behaviour of the anti-Levine majority, who shouted down those who wished to present reasonable arguments on the evening in question, was broadcast across Canada and proved an embarrassment to Ottawa.

This meeting became a turning point in a controversy that began on May 1, 1998, the day the appointment was announced. It encouraged some prominent politicians to speak out on behalf of Levine. It evoked a strongly critical response from Quebec, and a desire on the part of federalists for damage control. Many who had gone on record as opposing the selection of David Levine felt called upon to dissociate themselves from the behaviour and attitude of the mob. How can we account for a display of mob psychology that is so at odds with the stereotype of the phlegmatic English character?

The Levine affair began with the appearance of the *Ottawa Citizen's* May 1 front-page headline "PQ's envoy to head hospital," and the sub-heading "Ottawa Hospital chief once ran as candidate for separatist party." This immediately defined David Levine's separatist activities, not his professional qualifications, as the public's primary concern. Of course, when a newspaper chooses a particular headline to highlight an aspect of a story, there is always potential ambiguity. The newspaper can be emphasizing one or both of two different things: what it thinks will be of most interest to readers or what it thinks should be of most interest to readers. There is always a potential moral element in a paper's selection of emphasized facts. The upshot is that this headline encouraged readers who may not have done so to attach great importance to Levine's separatist past.

The *Ottawa Sun* had no story on Levine on May 1, though it did carry one on hospitals. Why no reference to Levine? The *Ottawa Citizen* had got the story ahead of time, making other media less inclined to give the story extensive coverage.[1] Later some media wrongly accused Levine of not being around to answer questions. In truth, he had been available at the May 1 press conference, but then went back to New York, where he was still delegate general for Quebec.

CFRA Radio picked up the story on the day of the announcement and ran a poll with its readers. In its City section, May 2, the *Citizen* reported: "About half of about 35 callers responding to a CFRA phone-in poll yesterday said Mr. Levine shouldn't be asked to renounce separatism. Some added that ability matters more than politics."

This poll should be compared to Lowell Green's later poll carried out on the morning of May 19, when the full impact of the media's treatment of Levine, including by Green himself, had occurred: 42–5 against Levine. Such a poll is of course unscientific; Green's audience, and still more those who actively respond, are likely to share his negative attitude. But the increase in anti-Levine feeling corresponds to my own assessment of what sentiments the *Citizen,* the *Sun* and CFRA were conveying in the period from May 1 to May 19.

Interest and emotion concerning David Levine's appointment peaked on two separate occasions. In Ottawa, the greatest influx of letters, phone calls, etc., according to both CFRA and *Ottawa Citizen* sources, came around May 15, the day Levine held a press conference in Ottawa. It was also the day that the *Citizen* wrote its City section editorial headed, in half-inch type, "David Levine should resign," and the *Ottawa Sun* likewise had an editorial headed "Resign." A slightly lesser peak came just after the May 19 meeting.

In Montreal French print media, and media across Canada, the story had a fairly low profile until the days following the raucous meeting of May 19, when the Ottawa Hospital board faced its critics. The meeting was followed by reaction from prominent politicians such as Jean Chrétien. This was met with further reaction, building to highest interest on May 22 and 23, just after the Ottawa Hospital board decided to stand by their decision to hire Levine. This is discussed in detail in Chapter Three.

Le Droit should be considered separately from the French media in Montreal. This Ottawa French-language newspaper gave the issue prominence from the start, with its front-page headline "Une tempête politique" ("A political storm") on May 2. The paper was alert to reports in the *Citizen* and later the *Sun*, and published direct criticism of letters, columns and editorials in those newspapers, as well as a mix of polemic and high-minded essays calling for civility. Unfortunately, only a small proportion of anglophones read *Le Droit*, so that its restraining influence was not very great.

The perception of Levine-as-separatist dominated public consciousness and was reinforced by feedback from a public already influenced by the *Ottawa Citizen* and Lowell Green's talk show. The *Ottawa Sun* was initially dormant.

As already suggested, perhaps it considered any story missed by its own newspaper and trumpeted by a competitor to be a non-story. Whatever the reason for the delay, the *Sun* soon underwent a sharp transformation, becoming the chief instigator and cheerleader of the anti-Levine forces. Starting May 18, the *Ottawa Sun* carried the Levine story on its front page for five consecutive days.

The Levine story lit the fire of public attention and fanned the flames to a high level of emotion. The kindling that kept the inferno raging was the legacy of raw emotions and fears created by health cutbacks under the Harris and Chrétien governments, fear about the future of Canada, about jobs, and the economic future of Ottawa-Carleton, perceived favouritism towards Quebec and francophones, and so on.

The story refused to die. Even after the hospital board made it clear on May 21 that it was sticking to its decision to hire Levine, regular stories on the issue still appeared: two former mayors back Levine;[2] a small group pickets the business of an Ottawa Hospital board member;[3] Levine has his first day on the job.[4] Two months afterward, allusions to the Levine affair were commonplace. It had entered the folk consciousness of the national capital region, at least.

Le Journal de Montréal, a newspaper congenial to separatist opinion, had a brief, informative story on May 7, followed by Michel Auger's column of May 15 and Pierre Bourgault's of May 18. By May 20, it identified the story as "L'Affaire Levine." The next day the story escalated into "Le Mouvement anti-Levine."

While the full attention of the Montreal French media began after May 19, there were earlier indications that Quebecers were noting what transpired in the English language media in Ottawa. On May 12 a statement was made in the House of Commons by the BQ member for Richelieu, Louis Plamondon, addressing the controversy about Levine's appointment in Ontario: "The whole episode involving Mr. Levine clearly shows that those who accuse sovereignists of creating ethnic divisions are in fact the ones who try to maintain such splits." On May 14 the first question was asked in the House by Bloc Québécois leader Gilles Duceppe, who again addressed the issue.

I shall examine the build up of concern as the David Levine affair began showing signs of becoming a national issue. What follows is a day-by-day analytical summary of events leading to the May 15 press conference.

Friday, May 1

Ottawa Citizen. Maria Bohuslawsky does what journalists are normally expected to do: start off with a good, attention-grabbing "angle." Her lead is "A former political candidate for the Parti Québécois is poised to become the president of the new amalgamated Ottawa Hospital." Levine's credentials are given no attention here. The idea that he might have been the most competent person available—a "catch," in professional terms—is not suggested. Although the newspaper does include an important biography, it is in a separate story done for the City section. By segregating the two stories a certain balance is lost.

Coincidentally I would assume, a photograph of a woman's anguished face is placed next to the story: a horrified Lara Rhodes, mouth open, hands holding her face. She is the wife of the Senators' hockey team goalie Damian Rhodes, and is shown reacting to the New Jersey Devils scoring against her husband. For those who felt aghast about a separatist or former separatist heading up the Ottawa Hospital, the picture gives a visual reinforcement of the feeling even though it is unrelated and facing away from the story.

The story gives a lot of factual detail. For example, it names eight of nine members of the hospital's search committee, and gives reasons why the committee had not placed much importance on Levine's separatist background. It also draws attention to the views of Ottawa-Rideau MPP Garry Guzzo, who objected to Ontario taxpayers supporting a Quebec separatist. "I'd want the board to be satisfied that his loyalties lie with Canada, and to the government that's paying his salary and not to a government whose goal [is] the breakup of this country," Guzzo is quoted as saying. In the following week, Guzzo will become a strident chief instigator of controversy and emotional protest.

Saturday, May 2

Ottawa Sun. The *Ottawa Sun*, perhaps disconcerted at having missed the big story on the previous day, comes out with a fairly prominent story emphasizing the defence of Levine and staking out ground opposite to the rival *Citizen* ("Hospital honcho defended" with a subhead "Separatist leanings of new CEO don't concern health officials"). It vents the views of an outraged Ottawa taxpayer and former Civic Hospital patient, and of an "incensed" MPP Garry Guzzo, who is quoted as saying that "the best person would be one who's committed to the Canadian flag." His view is contrasted with that of Michelle de Courville Nichol, chair of the board at the Montfort Hospital: "I have complete confidence in the board's selection." Of course, since the Montfort had been rescued from closure, and since it is a French-speaking hospital, this defence could easily be interpreted as adding fuel to the resentment against the appointment of a perceived pro-French administrator.

Le Droit. *Le Droit's* coverage, much more so than that of the *Ottawa Citizen*, gives a favourable impression of Levine. *Le Droit* emphasizes the views Levine himself had expressed about the opposition in the previous day's press conference: "I find it unfortunate. It's a storm over nothing. I was chosen by the selection committee because they were convinced that I could do the job and lead the hospital in the right direction. That's what interests me and it's a fascinating challenge for me." In support of the apolitical character of his hospital administration he said, "When I was named chief administrator of the Notre-Dame Hospital, in 1992, it was the Liberals who chose me for the job."

Ottawa Citizen. The important fact about his suitability to the Liberal government does not make its way into Joanne Laucius's story in the *Citizen.* Much later, on May 22, the *Citizen* runs a front-page banner headline proclaiming that "Levine was once a Liberal, too." It would have considerably dampened some of the fears about Levine had this information been presented to the English-language readership earlier. More space is taken up by the *Citizen's* story on Garry Guzzo, who received a hundred telephone calls at his constituency office and another sixty-five at his law office, mostly from irate residents. As time goes on the reported calls increase tenfold.

Monday, May 4

Ottawa Citizen and *Ottawa Sun.* On this day both the *Ottawa Citizen* and the *Ottawa Sun* carry editorials against Levine. The *Citizen's* is headed "Dubious choice;" the *Sun's* "Baggage." The *Citizen* editorial treats the appointment as "a cause of some concern" because Levine's PQ involvement meant that he "may not be the best person to deal with the touchy language issues facing the hospital." His close affiliation with a "group that has a history of mistreating anglophones" is seen as something that "may aggravate an already difficult situation." The editorial is embedded in a longer editorial on the problem of an inadequate supply of hospital beds for the elderly with long-term care needs ("Right idea, not enough beds").

Le Droit. Le Droit also provides some important biographical details: that Mr. Levine is president of the Canadian Association of Teaching Hospitals, that although he is perfectly bilingual he did not learn French before he was 24 or 25. He says that services in French would be "a priority for me" in the amalgamated Ottawa Hospital, as it is also a priority for the board that appointed him. He believes that the fears of francophones who were roused to preserve the Montfort Hospital were legitimate but that the Ottawa Hospital could offer a level of service in French equivalent to that in English. "We offer tertiary and quaternary services, so it is important that francophones can be treated in their language," he says.

Tuesday, May 5

Ottawa Citizen. Three letters, from W.A. Halliday of Orleans, Khoo Kim Lian of Fournier, and G.H. McGill of Nepean, are published prominently in the *Ottawa Citizen's* City section under the banner heading "Hiring separatist to run new hospital invites abuse." Halliday asserts that David Levine is a "tried, tested, true-blue, dyed in the wool (*pure laine*) separatist" and that taxpayers' money should not support someone who would further the PQ agenda: "I envision the abuse of public funds to support their position and to further their cause by several means. I can, for instance, see only francophones being hired at the hospital, and anglophone Ontarians being forced out to provide employment and salaries for closet separatists."

Khoo Kim Lian of Fournier (a village near Cornwall) laments that Canadians can't seem to distinguish friends from foes, and questions whether Levine has departed from involvement in politics. "David Levine was for the past year a PQ delegate general from Quebec to the United States. Yet he has been quoted as saying that he has not been involved in politics for well over 17 years and we take his word for it." She concludes by calling Levine a "traitor": "It seems that bilingualism is the most important qualification and we are willing to overlook the fact that this man is a traitor and would have been dealt with accordingly in any other country."

G.H. McGill refers to Levine as an "enemy" likely to turn the Ottawa Hospital into a Quebec-style hospital. "Look for the Civic and the General being equipped with French-first signage and French staff. It is hard to tell if you are in Ontario when you approach and enter the General."

The language of these letters is provocative, and flies in the face of tolerance. There is no moderating expression from the *Citizen* editorial corner.

Ottawa Sun. Interestingly, there are no letters either today or for the rest of the week in the *Ottawa Sun*. The only news coverage in the *Sun* had stressed points favourable to Levine. The editorial mentioned earlier, "Baggage," was negative.

Le Droit. *Le Droit* has an editorial by Paul Gaboury headed, "The 'sovereignist' CEO," which looks at those who mount the barricades against the Levine appointment and the overall implications for Canada. These people should ask themselves whether their behaviour is not more worrisome for the future of this country than Levine's separatist connections. Their outburst, writes Gaboury, "resembles a kind of paranoia having little connection with reason." In a mocking way, the editorial asks, "Does Mr. Guzzo fear the hospitals will be moved to Quebec? Are they afraid [Levine] will sell PQ membership cards in the hospital?" Gaboury notes that MPP Guzzo had proposed to lay off nurses from Quebec ahead of Ontario nurses. Guzzo should go to anglo hospitals in Quebec to see how they are pampered (*choyés*). The Franco-Ontarians don't know whether they can count on a single, open French hospital in Ontario, Gaboury writes.

Wednesday, May 6

Ottawa Citizen. The *Citizen* again devotes much space for letters, about 24 column-inches, with a three-line, half-inch headline "Hospital board must reconsider hiring president." All three letters are opposed to Levine's appointment. The first, by Stuart Busat, challenges the view that the hospital position is apolitical: "David Levine claims political opinions don't play a role in this appointed position. In my opinion, in Canada the issue of language is very much in the realm of political opinion, so his stated commitment to ensure French in all services is a stated political opinion." Busat believes Levine's political past "makes him unsuitable for this position as the location is too close to the border with Quebec." He also thinks Levine lacks "a network base in Ontario that would make him effective immediately in dealing with this institution's amalgamation." He urges the 32-member board not to ratify the appointment. What this letter doesn't mention is that the policy on language matters is a decision for the hospital board, not the CEO. Also, as David Levine saw in Montreal, having a network base can be a disadvantage. Having headed the Notre Dame Hospital, he did not appear impartial in relation to the other two hospitals to be amalgamated and this was the reason given for not choosing him to head the new hospital there.

Roughly speaking, people who write letters to newspapers fall into two classes: those who like to write letters and have a selection of causes that they wish to promote (This is an honourable activity, and those who do so often enrich the cultural life of a community.); and those who don't normally write but are stung sufficiently by a particular occurrence that they feel impelled to express themselves publicly. I contacted Stuart Busat by telephone and from hearing his background he seemed to me to fall into the latter class. He is originally from Montreal and worked for ten years as a night auditor at St. Mary's Hospital, the English Catholic Hospital. He found his career path blocked in Montreal following the election of the Parti Québécois in 1976. He had succeeded in obtaining a BA at Concordia, followed by an FBA and MBA. At St. Mary's he was told that his French was not good enough to allow him to occupy a senior position. So he started up his own business. But again people, both anglophones and francophones, questioned him about his lack of knowledge of French. So eventually after some frustrating experiences, he decided to move to Ottawa, where he now manages a business. In my early June conversation with Mr. Busat he was quick to dissociate himself from the intolerance expressed at the May 19 meeting, and regretted if in any way his letter had contributed to that spirit. He stressed that he was not anti-French, and could understand the motives of Quebecers who wanted to promote French in their own territory. What he wanted to avoid was the same kind of career blockage in Ottawa that he had experienced in Montreal.

In his letter to the *Citizen* George Potter of Fournier expresses apprehension that an avowed separatist would be given such a responsible position in Ontario. He fears there will be increased use of French with Levine in control: "[H]ow soon can we expect qualified anglophone staff to be replaced by less-qualified, bilingual francophones? And how much of the overall service will be in French for the majority anglophone patients?" Potter falls into the first category of letter-writer. His card reads "George Potter, Political Activist." A retired military man, first in Britain and then in Canada with the RCAF, he writes well-edited, strongly worded letters on a regular basis to a wide variety of media outlets and to politicians such as Premier Mike Harris and Prime Minister Jean Chrétien. His letters are often published in the *Citizen* and sometimes in out-of-the-way newspapers. He will occasionally fax letters to nine different newspapers. He has contacts with the Alliance for the Preservation of English in Canada (APEC), and says it is quite possible that a friend from Ottawa would have faxed him the news story from the *Citizen* that occasioned his letter. Among his causes are a desire to stem the immigration of gypsies from the Czech Republic, and the discouragement of gay sexual practices, without disparaging gay persons themselves. He recognizes that in the minds of some people he will be dismissed as a "crank," but feels it is important to swim against the tide sometimes. He believes that the anglophone minority in Quebec has undergone discrimination. He stresses that his wife is French-Canadian, that he is not anti-French and that his wife and daughter speak French at home.

The third letter "Wrong priority" is by Pauline Leitch of Thornhill. She begins by noting that the board would presumably have sought a bilingual individual to head the new Ottawa Hospital. "This helped put Mr. Levine at the head of the list. In a predominantly English-speaking hospital, bilingualism should not be a criteria *(sic)* for a president, particularly when the francophones have their own hospital, the Montfort." Her feeling is that the Montfort (French) Hospital had been slated to close, but political protest kept it open. She objects to Levine's statement that he is "very committed to ensuring the francophone community has all the services in their language" because, since the "overwhelming majority" of patients in the Ottawa area will be English-speaking, the administration should be English. She issues a call to arms to readers: "It wasn't Quebecers who reinstated our present dictator, it was Ontario. He is in your debt. Call in your markers. Make a big fuss! Don't let up. If this outlandish appointment is allowed to stand it will inevitably be followed by more of the same. Look what has happened to our military. Look at the disarray of the public service." She concludes with an observation that French language ranks fourteenth in worldwide usage while English ranks first. "If you don't stand up for your language, your culture, you not only will find yourselves second-class citizens, you'll deserve it." Since Pauline Leitch's address is in the Toronto area, one might raise the question how would she have seen the newspaper report about Levine. The answer is that she is married to Ronald P. Leitch, president of APEC. He explained to me that this kind of material (the May 1 Levine article) is often faxed to him by members.

The tone, quantity and length of the letters opposing Levine combine to create a sense of strong and widespread feeling against the appointment. None of the letters so far have supported Levine. The next day, in the *Citizen,* it is the same.

A newspaper's editorial position is easily influenced by articulate, informed letter writers. Robert Escarpit, the prominent French professor and media expert who was on faculty at the University of Bordeaux when I was there on sabbatical in 1979–80, once explained to me how he proved this theory. He and some prominent friends decided to write on a particular issue of the day upon which a newspaper had taken a position. They would contradict the newspaper's editorial position, but each one with his own separate, carefully expressed argument. They wrote from different parts of the country, so that the editor would not suspect collusion. Sure enough, when the letters had been received and assessed, the editorial position of the newspaper was promptly changed.

The moral is twofold. First, it is not common for well informed people to bother to write to newspapers to correct errors. Time is too short. So if someone who is clearly knowledgeable and articulate does bother to write, it makes an impact. When three such people write about the same matter, reflecting the same view, it has a powerful impact, so long as there is no suspicion of collusion. Second, the Escarpit example shows how vulnerable an unsuspecting editor can be to opinion that has organized assistance without being an obvious letter-writing campaign. Editors can easily get a disproportionate sense of how widespread and strongly held the ideas reflected in a sampling of letters may be among the public generally.

The informal links generated by APEC and at least one other organization formed to preserve the Civic Hospital may have given a somewhat distorted impression to the relevant editors about the kind of opinion held by the general public. Readers also tend to see public opinion as reflected in letters published. The exceptions are off-the-wall letters that sometimes find their way into print when the editor's aim is clearly to provoke and elicit rebuttals. Otherwise, a plurality of letters favouring a particular view gives the impression that a sizeable portion of the population holds the view. The effect of a succession of anti-Levine letters will have encouraged the belief that this is a fairly widely-shared opinion, and so have encouraged others to think along similar lines.

Le Droit. *Le Droit* takes note of the letters published in the *Ottawa Citizen* on May 5. A story by Denis Gratton comments on the "numerous letters" and quotes from the letters by Halliday, Lian and McGill, leaving out the bit about the "punishment for traitors" in Lian's letter. Gratton has interviewed Brian Sarjeant, letters editor of the *Citizen*, and comments that the *Citizen* has received more than twenty such letters and is going to publish three more today. He quotes Sarjeant: "They're all more or less the same. But I'll admit that some of them make me a bit uneasy. Like those of Mr. Potter, who writes to us regularly." Sarjeant felt sure that, as usual, there would be several calls from francophone readers offended by Potter's letter.

Thursday, May 7

Ottawa Citizen. Seven letters, somewhat shorter than the previous day's, are published in the City section of the *Citizen* under the two-column, three-line heading "Hiring separatist as hospital chief insults Ontarians." Six letters are against the appointment. Only one, published last, shows aversion to the dominant anti-Levine mood. The first, by Joe Pelisek of Gloucester is in response to the May 2 article, "Hospital appointment draws fire." He implies that Levine's reported priority of merging English and French cultures would favour the French: "If anyone who has any doubt, in spite of all kinds of assurance otherwise, just what that will eventually mean in terms of jobs, management, influence, etc., then they should book the first flight to the moon, leaving tomorrow."

Eva Brown of Kanata expresses her disbelief that "a former member of the Parti Québécois could even be considered for such a high position. "Is there not one single person in all of Ontario who could fill this position?" she asks. Frank T. Laverty of Ottawa views the appointment of an "avowed separatist" as "an insensitive insult to Ontarians who are federalist" and calls for immediate rescinding of Levine's appointment. W.G. Anderson of Nepean describes David Levine as being a "hard-core separatist" since the early '70s. "Now we have the fox in the henhouse—and a very comfortable fox at $300,000 annually. They must be rolling on the floor laughing out loud in the Bouchard Bunker." The reference to "hard-core separatist" presupposes a constancy in Levine's political affiliations that was later put into question. But repetition of such expressions, including Lowell Green's use of the term "rabid separatist" in his CFRA talk show, lend an air of truth to the notion, which later evidence showed was not the case.

R. Keith Plowman of Carleton Place describes the selection subcommittee responsible for recommending Levine as "incompetent." Don Ludlow of Kanata says that the board of trustees showed "poor judgement" in their choice. "Regardless of his professional qualifications, Mr. Levine has had longstanding and prominent connections with a political party whose avowed aim is the break-up of Canada and whose treatment of the Quebec anglophone minority has been less than generous," he writes.

The one letter favouring Levine is from Nepean resident Douglas Ruby, who writes: "It is lamentable that some people oppose David Levine's selection to head the Ottawa Hospital for political reasons. With the justified worries over the state of health care in Ontario, it is not in the best interests of the people of Ottawa-Carleton to choose anything less than the most qualified candidate." Ruby describes himself as a former Montrealer from the same community as Levine. He told me in an interview that the idea of Levine as a committed separatist did not fit well the image he had formed of him in Montreal. This was one example among many pro-Levine letter writers who were to appear much later.

Le Journal de Montréal. May 7 marks the first appearance of the Levine issue in *Le Journal de Montréal.* Though the newspaper's general tone is nationalist, it takes no note of the brouhaha developing in Ottawa; it is written from a Montreal-centred perspective. This insightful piece by Michelle Coude-Lord notes that the former director of Notre Dame Hospital, David Levine, was rejected for the chief administrative post of three large newly amalgamated Montreal university hospitals (the Notre-Dame, Hôtel-Dieu and Saint-Luc) and chosen for the amalgamated Ottawa Hospital. "It is not good for Quebec, but it is good for Ontario," was the word heard in corridors, she reports. Coude-Lord's report goes on to say that Levine had been rejected in Montreal for political reasons—though the official explanation was that he was too closely associated with the Notre-Dame Hospital. Quebec Health Minister Jean Rochon and the president of the hospital board, Jacques Girard, preferred Cécile Cléroux, who had no experience in health administration, said Coude-Lord. Her nomination was strongly contested by doctors and unions. "Nothing works any more," she wrote. "As for Mr. Levine, a recognized péquiste, he was given the post of Quebec envoy in New York as a consolation prize. But now he can go back to his only and true passion, hospital administration."

The story seems plausible, that Levine was a victim of political in-fighting in Montreal, lost out and relied on his friends in the PQ to bail him out. This story contrasts sharply with the thinking that seems to have seized some of Levine's Ottawa opponents; that Levine is a key player in Quebec Premier Lucien Bouchard's Machiavellian plot to promote separatism. Either Levine succeeds in promoting French, or he fails because of opposition, which will prove to Quebecers that they are unwelcome outside Quebec and that an autonomous Quebec is the only solution for the future.

Michelle Coude-Lord's account credits David Levine's skill at hospital administration, which is how one would perceive him if one had any confidence in the judgement of the Ottawa Hospital board. As a regular reporter on the hospital scene, she would probably have been attuned to the possibility of some Machiavellian funny business, had there been any. At this early stage in the Levine affair there is no hint of anything other than a straightforward desire on Levine's part to seek the kind of job that most interests him. As the drama plays out in the weeks to come, this version of events will fit well with what was to transpire.

Le Droit. Denis Gratton has another story in *Le Droit*, this time about Bloc Québécois member, Louis Plamondon, who has questioned the *Ottawa Citizen's* editorial policy regarding publication of letters by people outraged at the Levine appointment. It is uncalled for to publish letters that claim David Levine is "a separatist," "a traitor" and "an enemy of Canada," or that he would "hire only francophones to throw the anglophones out of work," Plamondon is quoted as saying. In Plamondon's view the letters represent a very small minority in

English Canada. He welcomes Levine as one who understands very well the reality of linguistic minorities.

Friday, May 8

Ottawa Citizen. The front page of the *Ottawa Citizen* gives further momentum to the anti-Levine tide. The story by Randy Boswell, one column at the bottom left of the page, is headed "New voice in chorus vs. Levine." It quotes local Carleton–Gloucester Liberal MP Eugène Bellemare as saying he was "disappointed" that Levine had been appointed. He acknowledged that hiring committees would be "treading on dangerous ground" if they probed the political background of every candidate, but he said that someone with a separatist background would normally be "persona non grata" in Ottawa-Carleton and other federalist regions.

The story goes on to say how Bellemare had dissociated himself from Garry Guzzo on other occasions, such as when Guzzo proposed in 1996 that Outaouais workers should be the first to be laid off when spending cuts came. Guzzo's anti-Levine view appears less intolerant now that it is shared by Bellemare, who opposed a hard-line response to Quebec in the past.

The story concludes with quotations from Guzzo, who is reported as saying that Levine would likely fill "the whole administration with separatists" as he "begins to hire his own staff." "It's more than Levine now. The entire administration is going to have a political agenda to break up this country." Guzzo's related worry was that the appointment would cripple fund-raising efforts.

These comments are extremely prejudicial and, to the extent that Guzzo is taken seriously, damaging to Levine. What evidence does Guzzo have for making these allegations, which constitute grounds for dismissal. The Regional Municipality of Ottawa-Carleton Employee code of conduct, states: "To ensure public trust in the RMOC, employees must be, and appear to be, both politically impartial and free of undue political influence in the exercise of their duties." It is surprising that the *Citizen* is prepared to leave Guzzo's remarks unchallenged. Right or wrong, most people assume that when elected representatives speak out they have some factual basis for what they say. Guzzo's allegations conflict markedly with the impression conveyed by Michelle Coude-Lord on the previous day. It's the kind of judgement that encourages hysteria.

With the endorsement of a Queen's Park MPP, a federal MP and Regional Councillor Betty Hill's comment in the *Citizen,* May 1, that the selection of Levine was "dangerous," the anti-Levine forces gained considerable momentum.

The *Citizen* carries five more letters, prominently placed in the City section page under the heading "Imagine Quebec hiring Reformer to run a hospital." Peter M. Jones of Gloucester writes: "Imagine a member of the Reform party, a former candidate currently employed as a trade commissioner in London for an English-speaking province, being hired to head a major hospital complex in Quebec." There would be a deluge of outrage and the appointment would not happen. "However, the appointment of David Levine gets no comments from our politicians. I can't understand why we continue to pay traitors from the public purse, and I consider all members of the Bloc Québécois and the Parti Québécois to be traitors because they advocate the destruction of this country." Once again repetition of the word "traitors" gives currency to this way of viewing separatists, though the official recognition accorded the BQ and PQ belies such a view.

A fairly lengthy but important letter by Marc Villemaire of Orléans defends the right of francophones to be served in the French language by public institutions. It argues against the letters of George Potter and Pauline Leitch, published May 6. Villemaire describes how as a Franco-Ontarian he did not feel at home in Quebec. He indicates that although the Montfort was preserved, it doesn't provide all needed services: "When the Sisters of Charity established the Ottawa General Hospital, one of their priorities was to serve the francophone community of Eastern Ontario. It was only after the General moved to its new location that there was a significant decline in French services. Although the Montfort will stay open, it will not continue to be a full-service hospital. Francophones do suffer heart attacks and strokes, we do need cancer treatment, and we have a right, when our life is at stake, to be served in our language, especially in an area where we form a significant part of the population." Villemaire says he accepts some of the concerns about the appointment of a separatist, but that service in French in a public institution is a very different matter.

A letter by David H. Boon and Frances Boon of Ottawa, headed "Amazing insensitivity," directs attention to David Levine's former New York job, describing it as one that promotes the division of Canada. The letter states that Levine has "refused to disassociate himself from the separatist goal of the breakup of Canada," and that he thus would be welcome back to the separatist fold when his contract ends. "This Ontario family deeply resents the taxes that we will pay towards Mr. Levine's $330,000 per annum salary and deplore (*sic*) the fact that we have been saddled by the hospital board of trustees with an anti-Canadian administrator for the contractual period."

Another letter by Ottawa's Lois Daley Laycock draws attention to Levine's Jewishness and wonders how he could support the separatists when Jacques Parizeau publicly put the blame for the recent PQ election defeat on the rich and ethnic groups. The letter inflates fears already expressed into the improbable claim that "We can now expect all employees in this new Ottawa hospital to be francophones, which will result in the exodus of our good doctors and nurses."

A final letter, by Joe Houlden of Gloucester, sees the concerns about bilingualism as applicable also to the advent of local, one-tier government, and he asks how the proponents of the mega-city planned to deal with the francophone element.

SATURDAY, MAY 9

Ottawa Citizen. Today the *Citizen's* coverage veers away somewhat from the heavily anti-Levine pitch adopted thus far. Previously, news, letters and editorials empowered the anti-Levine movement. On this day the *Citizen* publishes an eloquent, informative response from Nick Mulder, chair of the Ottawa Hospital board, concerning the reasons for hiring Levine. The headline, "An outstanding candidate," takes up four columns with half-inch type. Mulder explains that Levine was among sixteen candidates chosen by an internationally-respected search firm of Korn-Ferry after a search across Canada. A bilingual anglophone from Montreal, he had previous experience running the Verdun Hospital and subsequently Notre Dame Hospital in Montreal. Mulder also invites citizens in the community and region to attend meetings of the board to "learn more about their new hospital and to stay abreast of the progress and evolution of this vitally important institution." What he writes about the professional respect accorded Levine dovetails well with the *Le Journal de Montréal* story by Michelle Coude-Lord but *Citizen* readers would not likely have read that. Mulder's defence of the hospital's decision is an important move to counter the anti-Levine tide, but he is in a rhetorically weak position. People who are strongly anti-Levine already blame the hospital board and Mulder in particular. What Aristotle described as ethos, the character and credibility of a speaker, is low and carries little weight with those who have already made up their minds against Levine.

Two other letters follow Mulder's. Gérard Laurin, a retired public servant from Hull, draws attention to what he sees as the "hate and intolerance" that the reaction to Levine's appointment has revealed in the national capital. "It reminds me of a scene in the movie *Dances with Wolves* where the hero is severely punished for fraternizing with the Indians." In his view the Montfort Hospital, "the only solution for health services in French for francophones, has been virtually dismantled." He fears that with all the uproar, the stage has been set for self-censorship among those who would like to defend francophone rights: "Let us not exaggerate or confuse the issues for a few hate letters."

Finally, two Ottawa physicians, George Tolnai and Susan Tolnai, write to explain the great difficulties ahead with amalgamation of the hospitals. They conclude: "We should do everything possible to ease the difficult transition to an amalgamated hospital; elimination of a separatist from Quebec to the president's position would be a step in the right direction."

SUNDAY, MAY 10

Ottawa Citizen. More fuel for anti-Levine feeling hits the pages of the *Citizen* with a lengthy story, 50 column inches, by Kelly Egan under the heading "Levine still backs PQ: former MNA," and the subhead, "New head of Ottawa Hospital was member of commission to study Quebec sovereignty." Reed Scowen, a former Liberal MNA in Quebec, says that the job of delegate general to New

York was clearly a political one. As a previous holder of the same job, he had resigned the day that Jacques Parizeau became Quebec's premier. The third paragraph states that "Mr. Levine recently told the *Citizen* he's had no involvement with politics for 17 years." But this was followed with a contrasting view from Reed Scowen, that "any person who holds the job clearly has the premier's blessing."

The upshot of the story is to discredit Levine in the mind of the average reader. The impression is that he has not been candid in denying recent involvement in politics. That impression is further strengthened by the disclosure that Levine had been named to a "high-profile task force [in 1991] looking at the status and role of anglophones within a sovereign Quebec." He "was also a member of a commission set up by the PQ government in 1995 to gather input from Montrealers on the government's draft sovereignty bill." The story acknowledges that this was a "broadly-based group, with many political stripes," but notes that the "Quebec Liberal party and many federalists went so far as to boycott the commission." MNA David Payne, described as Premier Lucien Bouchard's "pointman for anglophone affairs" does not recall Levine as having a formal role in the 1991 task force and takes offence at the idea that someone might be impugned for having beliefs in line with a democratic political party. "Hey, what is this, a McCarthy hunt or something?" he asks reporter Kelly Egan. What this evidence amounts to is simply that Levine was willing to cooperate with the separatist government, not that he actively supported a "breakup of Canada," as his critics insist. The story concludes with the observation that "Mr. Levine has refused to disclose whether he holds separatist views."

Ottawa Sun. The *Ottawa Sun* carries one letter from Austin B. Tetley of Smiths Falls. He views the appointment of Levine as "completely out to lunch." "We should make our voices loud and clear, get rid of him with no separation bonus," he writes.

In running successive stories that suggest that David Levine is a separatist, the media, consciously or unconsciously, reinforce a certain subtext: that this separatist involvement is very important and that it does indeed make a big difference to Levine's suitability for the CEO position in the Ottawa hospital. And although that subtext should be directly questioned, it is simply assumed to be true.

Monday, May 11

Ottawa Citizen. A column in the City section of the *Citizen*, headed "Hospital president owes us answers," by Susan Riley, keeps up the attack on the Levine appointment, although she balances this with criticism of Garry Guzzo's claim that Levine would "fill the whole administration with separatists." This statement is "simply irresponsible and absurd," she writes, but coming three days after the *Citizen* printed the original remarks, the impact of her words is somewhat lessened. She also adds: But "[i]t is reasonable to ask if, in our earnest effort to be fair, Canadians aren't sometimes foolishly generous."

Riley's emphasis is on the aversion to Levine's political beliefs, and the need for a "full accounting of his political views and his ambitions for the hospital." She says nothing about the abilities that might make him a particularly good candidate. Although she mentions the guarantee of freedom of belief in the Canadian Charter of Rights and Freedoms, she seems to think that disclosure of belief is nevertheless owed to the people when the demand for disclosure is not based simply on "mere prejudice." The upshot of her column is that there was probably no choice but to accept the appointment, but people don't have to like it.

The *Citizen* letters section gives prominence to two letters criticizing health services under the heading "Nurse shocked by poor service at Civic Hospital." Neither of the letters has any reference to David Levine, but indirectly they contribute to a sense of concern about the person appointed to run the new hospital. Three letters about the Levine affair appear under the heading "Appointment of separatist fuels English-only rants." The first letter, by Frank Howard of Ottawa, uses strong language in calling for reversal of Levine's appointment: "Mr. Levine has cast his lot, on more than one occasion, with those who proposed for fun and profit that our country could be tossed aside like a used nose-wipe. Let him find work with that gang again." Howard also criticizes the decision for the likely effect it will have on resuscitating the Association for the Protection of English (perhaps meaning the Alliance for the Preservation of English in Canada), which he links with those "English-only nuts who see the appointment as part of a conspiracy to force French down their throats."

Howard's vindictiveness towards separatists and stereotyped view of their attitudes overlooks the fact that people like Levine were originally attracted to separatism's socially progressive philosophy on economic matters. He also ignores Levine's abilities to manage the complicated process of hospital amalgamation with curtailed funds. Avoidance of this issue conforms to *Citizen* coverage up to this time.

Robert C. Cross of Renfrew notes that in light of the groundswell of opinion against Levine, twelve *Citizen* letters against and only one for, Levine should resign or his appointment be rescinded.

A final letter by Norman Bobitt of Lac Ste-Marie, Quebec, voices concern about the "diatribe of anti-French letters appearing in the *Citizen*." He defines two kinds of separatists who are basically in agreement: One wants Quebec to be separate; the other is in effect telling the separatists to go back to Quebec, as they are not welcome in Ontario.

Ottawa Sun. As already mentioned, the *Ottawa Sun* ignored the Levine issue for a full week, but its May 11 edition carries as the main headline "Heart doc crisis," a reference to a feared shortage of cardiac surgeons within six years. Also covered is Quebec Premier Lucien Bouchard's slight to the memory of former Prime Minister Mackenzie King when he unveiled a monument to the Quebec City conference of Roosevelt and Churchill that left out Mackenzie King. This adds more fuel to anti-separatist feeling.

Le Droit. Le Droit has a very witty cartoon. A photograph of a smiling Levine is shown surrounded by excerpts from letters published in the *Citizen*, such as "We are willing to overlook the fact that this man is a traitor and would have been dealt with accordingly in any other country" and "Look for the Civic and the General being equipped with French first signage and French staff. It is hard to tell if you are in Ontario when you approach and enter the General." Levine is saying, "There are more sick people than I anticipated."

On the opposite page Denis Gratton's column attacks Carleton-Gloucester Liberal MP Eugène Bellemare's remarks, which were quoted in the *Citizen* on May 8. "So what?!" about Levine's separatist affiliations, he says. Gratton denies being a separatist, but says he understands those who are: "Because they want more or less the same as us: the right to live in French; the right to flourish in their language; the respect of their language and culture." To the argument that they want to break up the country, he replies: "No. They want to give themselves a country. Nuance." In Gratton's view, "The only way to keep Canada united is to hold out a hand to Quebecers and not to spit in their face."

Tuesday, May 12

Ottawa Citizen. Today the *Citizen* news story, on page three of the City section, is much more favourable to Levine than hitherto. The headline to Maria Bohuslawsky's story is "Hospital president's task 'apolitical'" and the subhead states "'David Levine's political sympathies don't matter,' surgeon says." Dennis Pitt, a general surgeon at the Riverside Hospital and head of the Academy of Medicine of Ottawa, is quoted as saying that most local doctors regard Levine's PQ background as irrelevant. The administrator has a "relatively apolitical task. It really doesn't matter what his political sympathies are," he said, "Some (hospital workers) are very, very redneck. Some of them are way right of the Reform party in their attitudes, but this has nothing to do with the way they function professionally." The story also draws attention to Regional Councillor Alex Munter who would like to see the election of board members by the general public and who objected to the hospital board's lack of accountability to the electorate.

In the City letters section two letters oppose Levine's appointment under the banner headline "Defence of Ottawa Hospital CEO avoids key issue." Bob Jones of Nepean denies that "hate and intolerance" motivate his opposition; that it is Levine's separatism, not his professional qualifications, that are behind the public reaction; and that Levine is connected to "a political party that wants to break up this country." According to Jones, Garry Guzzo "even determined on May 8 that Mr. Levine had to swear an oath of allegiance to the separatist cause before taking on his current New York position at the behest of Premier Lucien Bouchard," although he does not name Guzzo's source. Much later, on June 9, the Ottawa Hospital will issue the statement: "Mr. Levine took no Oath of Allegiance since this was not a requirement of the job."

Jones feels that Ottawa Hospital chair Nick Mulder should have addressed the issue, and is perplexed that Levine, a member of the Montreal Jewish community, should support the separatists when his community felt under attack from them. He concludes by calling for a letter from Levine, or a public appearance, explaining his expectations for Canada. The Canadian Jewish Congress, Quebec region, later defended Levine's freedom of opinion and suitability for the job, as reported in *Le Devoir* May 19 ("Le Congrès juif déplore les réactions négatives.")

John Angus, in the second letter, wonders whether Levine's "separatist leanings are the result of unprincipled self-promotion and ambition" or whether Levine is "a blithering idiot." In neither case, says Angus, would Levine have the character traits that Ottawans have a right to expect from someone holding the job.

Ottawa Sun. In the *Ottawa Sun,* Dale Hibbard's letter attacks Ottawa-Gloucester MP Eugène Bellemare and Ottawa-Rideau MPP Garry Guzzo for their "asinine logic" in opposing Levine's appointment, saying that if it prevailed it would prohibit anyone from "being operated on by anyone other than a federalist surgeon." The *Ottawa Sun*, as is its customary practice, appends its own discourse-stopper: "Sorry, but we think they're right, you're wrong."

Wednesday, May 13

Ottawa Citizen. The Levine story is once again on the front page of the *Citizen*, though this time with a new basis for opposing Levine: "Outraged hospital donors protest Levine hiring." The lead paragraph reads: "Hundreds of outraged donors have vowed to stop supporting the Civic Hospital Foundation—with some ready to change their wills—to protest the appointment of a former Quebec separatist as chief of the region's new amalgamated hospital." The source is Tom Hewitt, executive director of the foundation, who said he had received 250 calls to protest the Levine appointment. The Civic Foundation reportedly raises between $4 million and $6 million each year for the Civic hospital site. Garry Guzzo is also reported as having been told by about 50 people that they would no longer support the hospital financially. Ellen Ewart, director of development for the Foundation of the Ottawa General Hospital, also had received more than a dozen calls from donors saying they will no longer pledge money to the hospital, the story says.

In the *Citizen's* City section columnist Randall Denley protests the lack of accountability of the hospital board to the general public. One solution he proposes is for regional councillors to take the responsibility for overseeing the system. On the letters page, the only letter in defence of Levine is given top place and the headline, "Political affiliation doesn't justify job discrimination."

Three other *Citizen* letters oppose the Levine choice. John Edwards of Ottawa observes that the appointment "precipitated a popular outpouring of anti-separatist sentiment." He affirms his commitment to Canada but says he is "very uncomfortable" at the idea that people should be screened from jobs "simply because they support or have supported sovereignist parties." He concludes on a very optimistic note: "As a long-time resident of this region, I am happy that the selection board had the courage to select the candidate whom they judged could do the job best. And if David Levine has still any separatist leanings, I am confident he will lose them as he grows to enjoy this tolerant and thoughtful city!"

Bill Armstrong quotes from a letter he sent to the Ottawa Civic Foundation: "Please remove my name from the list of donors to the foundation. I have lost all confidence in the board of directors of the Ottawa Hospital and my most effective means of protest is to withdraw my support from any agency connected with the Ottawa Hospital. The board has selected a CEO who has a serious conflict of interest. He has made it clear that his loyalty lies with Quebec. The Ottawa Hospital is an Ontario institution which also makes available services to citizens of Quebec. Someone who puts Quebec's interests first, whether currently politically active or not, cannot be an impartial CEO of an Ontario hospital."

The letter assumes that Levine's loyalty to Quebec would take precedence over his duty to Ontario and his professional concerns. This assumption has not been proven. In fact, counter-evidence is available, notably in the *Journal de Montréal* story of May 7, which was quoted earlier. The hospital board later makes it clear, in a June 9 statement, that "any attempt to bring political beliefs—no matter which party he is loyal to—into the job ... would be cause for the Board to terminate his contract."

In his letter, John Larivière raises another point of great importance that was to be repeated often, namely the frequent failure of Quebec to honour Ontario rates when Quebecers come to be treated in Ontario hospitals. "Language is never a problem for francophones in need of medical care that is not available in Quebec, or available there at lower standards than those provided in Ottawa," he writes. He concludes that Ontarians are concerned that Ontario taxpayers have to pay the difference between Ontario and Quebec rates, "despite the fact that Quebec acts in violation of our National Health Act." "We are also convinced that a hard-core Quebec nationalist of Mr. Levine's calibre will never open his mind to recognizing such a blatant injustice—one that illegally siphons subsidies out of Ontario health-care funds." As I will discuss later, this point is stressed by Dr. Charles Shaver. As I mentioned previously, what is not made clear is how this issue is pertinent to the decision to hire David Levine, since the dispute about payment is a matter for the Quebec and Ontario ministries to resolve, perhaps with pressure from the federal government. This point is affirmed in the hospital board's June 9 statement: the issue is "up to the provincial Governments, not the Board, to resolve and the Board hopes this will be done as soon as possible." Those hostile to Levine seem to assume that he has powers, which he does not in fact have, to rectify the dispute about payments.

By this time the discussion has reached a point where a lot of people are thinking about the legal ramifications of terminating Levine's contract. Jim Redfern of Carleton Place thought that the Levine appointment should be nullified, and that if sued for breach of contract the board should be "held accountable for the offensive selection of an avowed enemy of a united Canada to preside over the primary health care facility in this area."

Thursday, May 14

It becomes clear by today that the Levine issue is not likely to blow over. Fund-raising problems take centrestage, and the Ontario Minister of Health makes a statement giving encouragement to the anti-Levine forces.

Ottawa Citizen. Once again the Levine story makes the front page of the *Citizen* with the headline "Levine protest gaining strength" and the subhead "Police veteran writes hospital out of will; health minister voices concerns." The lead paragraph recounts how retired police officer Robert Proulx has decided not to leave money to the amalgamated hospital as a result of the Levine appointment. Proulx clarifies that he is not against somebody from Quebec or somebody French, but someone who is separatist. "I have a problem with his political affiliations," he says. On the next page a 4 inch x 6 inch close-up photograph of a close-mouthed Proulx, with an extended hand bearing prominent rings on two fingers, gives emphasis to the story.

Ontario Health Minister Elizabeth Witmer is reported as saying that, although she would not intervene in Levine's appointment, the hospital board should consider the implications of his hiring: "The local hospital board obviously needs to take a look at the impact of this decision they made and they need to be giving it some very, very serious consideration themselves." This statement is not overlooked by some of the French-language media, who see this as a surrender to the anti-Levine forces and an abandonment of the principle of freedom of opinion.

A second headline appears on the front page of the City section: "Hospital director's Quebec links won't help Ontario physicians: doctor." In this Charles Enman story, Ottawa physician Charles Shaver is quoted as saying, "Where the Quebec government wants to pay lower than normal fees to the hospital and the doctors who work there you can be sure David Levine will have lots of time for Quebec interests." As mentioned earlier, however, provincial payments are a matter for the provincial ministerial level, and in any case the CEO must keep his political beliefs separate from the job. Shaver himself has faulted the federal government for not enforcing relevant provisions of the Canada Health Act.

The story provides useful information about medical fees arrangements among other provinces: "When a Quebec resident receives medical care in another province, the Quebec health plan pays only the fees for service that it pays to physicians practising in Quebec. All other provinces pay the usual fee for service of the host province. For example, if an Ottawa physician treats a New Brunswick patient for an eye injury, New Brunswick pays the normal fees established under the Ontario fee schedule. But if the patient is from Quebec, Quebec pays only what it would pay a physician practising in Quebec— and Quebec's fees are the lowest in the country."

The Quebec rate is reportedly about 30 percent lower than the Ontario rate. For West Quebec patients treated in an Ottawa Hospital the Quebec government will pay only $450 a day, whereas other provinces pay $745, the story says. Shaver claims there is "clear violation of the portability provision of the Canada Health Act." What the story did not say, but what Dr. Shaver told me in an interview, is that there is a special arrangement in the national capital region, whereby Quebec will pay the higher amount under certain circumstances. But complicated forms must be filled out, and there are many loopholes in the special arrangement, so that it often works out as if the arrangement did not exist.[5] Dr. Shaver also takes issue with Dr. Dennis Pitt (see May 12), saying, "I canvassed a good dozen of my colleagues at a meeting of cardiologists last weekend. Not one favoured Mr. Levine's appointment."

The story refers to Levine's New York appointment as one that "has been described as highly politicized and not a plum likely to fall into the hands of a federalist or tepid separatist." The phrase "has been described" does not indicate who does the describing; the reader is not assisted in evaluating the merits of the description by reference to the credentials of the person making the judgement.

Ottawa Sun. Finally on this day, the *Ottawa Sun* decides to engage again in Levine coverage, having ignored the story for nine days straight. In the days to come it will pursue the story with a vehemence unmatched by its rival *Citizen*. The *Sun* changes its position as a slight counter-weight to the *Citizen's* attack on Levine to become the leader of the attacking forces, with columnist Earl McRae providing bagpipe skirl and drumbeat.

Earl McRae uses the provocative language heard on the mouthier talk-in radio shows. Under the headline "Time for Levine to do the right thing," he opens: "The thundering stupidity of hiring David Levine does not need to be compounded by the thundering stupidity of David Levine refusing to resign as the inaugural chief executive officer of the newly amalgamated Ottawa hospital."

His argument hinges on the local community's perception of David Levine as a separatist and stirs up deep-seated opposition to use of taxpayers' money for supporting someone, no matter how qualified, who would be in a position to further the break-up of Canada. "Don't you get it, Levine? Don't you get it Mulder and company? How clueless are you anyway? This isn't about Levine's credentials as a hospital administrator. It's about *perception*. The perception, here, is more significant than any reality."

McRae goes on to compare the Levine affair to hiring an arsonist to be in charge of a fire hall: "The dry, kindling wood beneath the hot sun in this community, just waiting to be combust, is called French/English Sensitivities." His column concludes: "Pack it in, David Levine. And, if you won't pack him in, Nick Mulder and Gang of Fools, you can damn well pack yourselves in."

A news story on page 8 of the same paper further airs the views of Garry Guzzo, who finds it "disheartening" that Ontario's health minister, Elizabeth Witmer had remained silent on the Levine affair. "Guzzo's office has received more than 600 calls and 165 faxes or letters expressing outrage at the board's move." Guzzo is also quoted as saying: "When choosing the best qualified person for the job, one of the factors is a commitment to the flag of this country."

Le Devoir. *Le Devoir* columnist Graham Fraser writes a very informative column on the Levine affair ("Nomination scandale à Ottawa"), placing emphasis first on Levine's qualifications as an expert on hospital amalgamation, having served from 1992 to 1997 as director general of the Notre-Dame Hospital in Montreal when it was amalgamated with Saint-Luc and Hôtel-Dieu; prior to that he was head of the Verdun Hospital for ten years. He goes on to quote Nick Mulder's highly positive assessment of Levine's fitness for the post: "He has a national profile and a reputation as a leader .... His many professional activities include a term as president of the Canadian Association of Teaching Hospitals."

"Why then the opposition to Levine?" Fraser asks. In answer, he cites Levine's separatist connections, including his term as advisor to Bernard Landry in 1977 and his nomination by Jacques Parizeau to the commission on sovereignty. Because he refused to say that his position on separatism has changed, people have denounced him rather than welcoming him as a prodigal son, Fraser writes. He quotes Garry Guzzo as predicting that Levine would fill the hospital with separatists: "The entire administration will have a political agenda to destroy the country." To this Fraser replies: "What stupidity ... as if there were a separatist or federalist way of running a hospital! Come on!" These remarks, Fraser says, are the calculated opinions of politicians, which are distinct from comments of a less thoughtful nature on radio and in newspapers. On the basis of the latter he rightly predicts a turbulent meeting the following Tuesday, May 19.

Fraser thinks that the deep anti-separatist bitterness revealed in the Levine affair indicates a disturbing polarization. Hitherto he had sometimes thought that English Canada would react in a rational way to Quebec independence, once it had taken place. He now sees a real possibility of destructive behaviour, despite the phlegmatic and pragmatic reputation of the English.

This day, May 14, also marks the first mention of David Levine in the House of Commons question period, thus affording us an opportunity to compare later news accounts with the debate as officially recorded in Hansard. Bloc Québécois leader Gilles Duceppe refers to a statement made by Minister of Intergovernmental Affairs Stéphane Dion that "As long as there is threat of separation, this kind of problem is to be expected," and asks whether Dion recognizes that "by the irresponsible remarks he made and keeps making, he is condoning and justifying the unacceptable behaviour of those who wish to take this position away from Mr. Levine simply because he once ran in an election under the sovereignist banner?"

Liberal Deputy Prime Minister Herb Gray sees an opportunity to take a poke at the separatist party: "Mr. Speaker, we ought to be pleased to see the leader of the Bloc suggest that the federal government interfere in an area wholly under provincial jurisdiction. What position will the Bloc take next in this House in support of the federal position? Are they turning totally against Quebec separating from the rest of Canada?"

Michel Gauthier, BQ from Roberval responds: "We are not asking the federal government to interfere. We are simply asking the Minister of Intergovernmental Affairs, who made some unfortunate statements, to give us an explanation. "Will the minister not admit that his ministerial responsibility is not to add fuel to the fire on an issue such as this one, but rather to strongly condemn those who want to prevent someone from getting a job because of his political beliefs?"

Under further pressure from Gauthier, Dion responds: "Mr. Speaker, if there is one thing in which I strongly believe, it is freedom of conscience. I strongly believe that politics should have no influence whatsoever on the public service. I would never ask anybody to take an oath of allegiance. But in the light of the threat of separation, we are lucky that this kind of problem is not as severe in Canada as it would be in other democracies."

Until now, the *Ottawa Citizen* and the *Ottawa Sun* have tipped the scales against Levine with coverage that on the whole portrays him as a separatist party faithful, bent on carrying on a political mission in Ontario. Instead of examining that portrayal for accuracy, Earl McRae has told his readers that the perception is what is really important, not the reality. How this "McRae doctrine" squares with respect to individual freedom of belief and association is not made clear. But the willingness to accept perception as reality sets in motion a self-perpetuating spiral. The angrier the demonstration against Levine, the stronger the *perception* that he should go, and thus the greater the justification for being angry when he does not, and so on.

NOTES

1. This story is told in detail in Chapter Five.
2. See Maria Bohuslawsky, "Former mayors praise Levine," June 25, 1998, C2. In the story former mayors Jacquelin Holzman and Jim Durrell praised David Levine after meeting with him. Although former mayor Marion Dewar had already defended Levine at the May 19 meeting, Holzman and Durrell could be expected to appeal to a section of anti-Levine opinion less amenable to persuasion by an NDP stalwart.
3. See, for example, Nathan Vardi, "Ramsay targeted for fourth day," (*Ottawa Citizen,* June 21, A14) a story about the picketing of board member Barbara Ramsay's Shopper's Drug Mart outlet at Merivale Mall. Also, "Group wants Levine to resign" and "Anti-Levine protesters picket another hospital trustee," in the *Citizen*, June 29, C2 and C8 respectively.
4. David Levine's first day on the job got front-page coverage in the *Ottawa Sun,* June 16.
5. Interview with Dr. Charles Shaver, June 29, 1998.

Chapter Two

Second Press Conference, May 15

At the press conference of May 15, David Levine was expected by many to disavow his separatist past. He chose not to address the issue, even though there were certainly indications that "rabid separatist" hardly characterized the pattern of his connection with the PQ. By his silence he was, in the minds of many people, acknowledging some truth in the charges against him. A more sophisticated interpretation would be that he was unwilling to concede that belief or lack of belief in separatism was a legitimate criterion for running the Ottawa Hospital. In any case, Levine's stance gave renewed vigour to the opposition and further fuelled the uproar of May 19. Here we consider the media coverage leading up to the May 19 meeting.

Friday, May 15

Judging by letters and telephone calls to the media, today and the next day mark a peak in the controversy in the Ottawa area, although the most attention-getting display of public feeling will be reserved for May 19. Everyone by now knows of David Levine, and on this day he will be giving a press conference to explain himself. Local CFRA talk-show host Lowell Green devotes his three-hour morning program to Levine (the fifth day in which he is the topic), including live coverage of the press conference. Both English language newspapers call for Levine's resignation.

Ottawa Sun. The *Ottawa Sun* carries a one-inch front-page headline in bold: "Levine to 'set record straight.'" Many people expected him to renounce his separatist beliefs. Hospital board chair Nick Mulder is quoted as saying that Levine "believes in Canada." An unrelated photograph of Jerry Seinfeld, smiling and holding his thumb up, gives a sense of optimism, which rubs off onto the image of Levine conveyed in the main story. The *Sun's* news coverage as a whole, unlike the editorial and one of the letters, does not have a particular anti-Levine slant.

Another *Ottawa Sun* story on page 5, headed "Under the Microscope," reports that "[a]fter private talks, Mulder said he's satisfied Levine is not a separatist." It quotes Mulder: "He certainly is not committed to tearing up this country—not at all. He believes in Canada .... He may have had views at one stage or another—about the role of Quebec in Confederation, not so much separation."

44

An Ottawa Hospital worker, Brian Cayen, is reported as saying he would no longer raise money for the General Hospital Foundation if a separatist headed the hospital. In the previous year he had raised $1,250 for the foundation.

Scott Rowand, past president of the Canadian Teaching Hospitals Association is quoted as saying that Levine was one of only a handful of people in Canada with the background and experience to guide the Ottawa Hospital through the complicated merger. "His political views are completely irrelevant."

The *Ottawa Sun's* editorial, "Resign," takes the line that Levine would not be of much value to the hospital if he continues to be a "lightning rod for public anger and frustration": "Canadians are tolerant people. But even toleration has its limits." It holds Levine responsible for his political choice "albeit 20 years ago" and its repercussions: "Separatists can't mount a sustained campaign to denigrate Canada and all it stands for in Quebec and around the world and not expect that, once in awhile, Canadians will say enough is enough."

Although this statement does not directly accuse Levine of denigrating Canada, it imputes guilt for an association that took place twenty years ago. More pertinent evidence would stem from what Levine might have said or how his actions might have reflected a hostile attitude towards Canada. When I interviewed one of his associates in New York about Levine's activity there I uncovered no such attitude, though naturally he was concerned to advance the fortunes of Quebec. The fact that he was willing to leave Quebec for Ontario to pursue his main ambition of hospital administration should have indicated his favourable attitude towards Canada, but rumours carried by CFRA, as we shall see below, offset that presumption.

In a letter that outlines the most extreme of conspiracy theories, T. Conners attacks a previous writer, Dale Hibbard (May 12),[1] for referring to Levine as having "formerly" been an active Quebec separatist: "Give your head a shake. Levine has been appointed to further destroy this country only 'acting' as CEO of the new Ottawa Carleton board of directors." Such bold, unsubstantiated assertions are a hallmark of McCarthyism. In the spirit of Arthur Miller's *The Crucible*, Conners accuses Hibbard of being a separatist because he defended Levine, whose arrival is likened to a "new strain of 'cancer'" entering the hospital system—life threatening and needing drastic action. This strong and dangerous language, reminiscent of that used by Hitler in the 1930s, is an incitement to violence. And, when the *Ottawa Sun* ought to combat this dangerous language, it applauds it instead with the remark "Amen to that."

Ottawa Citizen. The *Ottawa Citizen* carries a friendly-looking 6 inch by 9 inch picture of Levine on the top of its front page, a suit draped over his arm, with the heading in three-quarter inch type, "Levine won't resign." The headline is based on a statement by the hospital board chair, Nick Mulder. The story, by Maria Bohuslawsky, Mark Gollom and Sharon Kirkey, is about his arrival to "confront concerns about separatist connection." The photo caption reads:

"Upon his arrival at Ottawa airport last night, former PQ candidate David Levine declined to reveal whether his commitment to separatism has changed." In the middle of the same page is a report of the previous day's parliamentary exchange between BQ leader Gilles Duceppe and Intergovernmental Affairs Minister Stéphane Dion, entitled "Furore akin to FLQ witch-hunt, Bloc says."

Inside, in the City section, a fourteen column-inch editorial calls for Levine's resignation. "David Levine should resign," proclaims the headline. Why? The public opposition will make him ineffective in his job. Donors are withdrawing contributions and volunteer time. "A prominent physician has publicly wondered whether Mr. Levine will act in the hospital's best interest in fee disputes with the Quebec government." Others object to a separatist being rewarded with a plum job. Even Ontario Minister Elizabeth Witmer had suggested the hospital board look seriously at the implications of the decision.

The editorial further holds it against Levine that "he has affiliated himself with a political organization that has a history of diminishing anglophones' rights." To say that it's unfair to deny a Canadian a job on the grounds he is a separatist would be "carrying evenhandedness to an extreme. Political sensitivities do matter." The situation is analogous to appointing a prominent member of the Alliance for the Preservation of English in Canada to run a hospital in Lac St. Jean. Even if highly qualified as an administrator, such a person would be a "poor candidate." "Unfortunately for Mr. Levine," the editorial continues, "his image in this community is not a positive one and that can only hurt his employer, the hospital." It says nothing about the *Citizen's* own role in shaping that negative image. The editorial concludes that Levine would be doing the best thing for Ottawa-Carleton and the Ottawa Hospital if he were to gracefully withdraw from the position. "Failing that, the board should dismiss him and bear the costs of doing so. The board says it's responsive to the public. The public has made its views quite clear. It's time to act before this error in judgement becomes more costly."

This editorial shows no awareness of the impact that the action it has counselled would have on Canada as a whole. What is remarkable is that the *Citizen* should appeal, in defence of its position, to a public attitude that it has had a substantial role in shaping. Later coverage proves to be more accepting of Levine's appointment, however, and this came to be reflected in the letters as well. This was the day on which Levine met with the *Citizen's* editorial board, winning over some though not all of its members.

The entire letters page is devoted to the Levine issue. Nine letters appear in total: three for, three against, and three of a neutral, questioning kind. Ron Crowley of Ottawa questions the composition and accountability of the hospital board, calling for a board policy statement from chair Nick Mulder and an assurance that Levine will remove himself from active politics while carrying out the board's policies.

Vivek Krishnamurthy, a high school student from Orléans, views the hospital post as apolitical and asks whether the federalist cause has "become so weak that it must resort to petty and mean-spirited personal attacks to keep Canada united?"

A third letter, from Dr. Charles Shaver, reiterates the points reported in the previous day's news story about Quebec's failure to pay Ontario full costs for treating its patients. Shaver's letter was the impetus for that story.

The fourth letter questions Nick Mulder's defence of the Levine appointment. Brian Seed of Ottawa writes that the defence missed the point, which was the "overridingly important question of the public's right to demand Mr. Levine's absolute loyalty and accountability to Canada and not to a separatist manifesto." His "past and present activities clearly raise serious questions about that essential point that can't be ignored."

A fifth letter, by Daniel Brunton of Ottawa, has its own headline in three-eighths inch type: "Levine's hiring 'sheer madness.'" It draws parallels between Levine's position and that of Brian Mulroney as chair of the National Capital Commission, Alan Eagleson as president of Sports Canada, and Don Cherry as Official Languages Commissioner. It argues that the new hospital CEO should have some empathy with his community and that more than technical expertise is involved. Accompanying photographs of Mulroney, Eagleson and Cherry give prominence to the letter.

Greg Gyton of Ottawa supports Levine, suggesting that people focus less on separatism and more on the issue of quality care in the new Ottawa Hospital. In commenting on his recent experience at the Civic hospital's emergency department he observes: "Many staff members seemingly working without direction, without motivation, without a sense of time, and (with a few exceptions) without much regard for the comfort or welfare of the patients. Imagine waiting for two hours with an excruciatingly painful broken foot before any sort of painkiller is offered. Imagine the wounded and elderly ignored and abandoned in the corridors, without so much as a glass of water." The challenge, says Gyton, "is to create measurable benchmarks for Mr. Levine to make the desperately needed improvements to the hospital's delivery of health care. I would much prefer the community to measure him on results rather than on policies."

Like Brian Seed, A.E. Spencer of Nepean thinks that Mulder had missed the point in his defence of Levine. "There is only one key issue," he writes. "Mr. Levine's political affiliates would see this wonderful country torn apart. This is a free country and Mr. Levine is entitled to his views but do we have to pay him for it? To pay this man $300,000-plus in Canadian dollars is unacceptable." Spencer intends to withhold donations to the hospitals until the "unacceptable" decision is reversed.

Ottawan Scott French writes that tolerance is generally good, but in the case of "blatant separatism," it is mistaken. Enough letters have been written, he says, to show that Levine's political views are indeed an issue. A "traitor," he said, "shouldn't be rewarded like this and people know it." He hopes that Levine will resign and a "more complex, more effective definition of tolerance" will be found.

Finally, a letter from Richard Fidler, identifying himself as one who favours sovereign status for Quebec, attacks Susan Riley for her May 11 column, on grounds that she showed a failure of imagination in seeing a contradiction between living in Ottawa and supporting Quebec sovereignty. "Quebec's accession to sovereignty will not necessarily harm Canada," he writes. It might even be "precisely the necessary first step to breaking the constitutional logjam and redefining a new association ... a true 'federation' in place of the current constitutional arrangement ...." He sees the real danger to Canada as coming from the "ongoing—and deepening—failure of the federalist imagination in English Canada and in the federal government." As an aside, he notes that Quebec protects political beliefs in its human rights code, unlike Ontario.

French Press. On May 15 the French press gives serious attention to the issue. *Le Droit's* front-page story, "Levine wants to clear the air" ("Levine veut faire le point"), simply describes some of the opposition to Levine, mentioning MPP Garry Guzzo in particular. Another story on page two quotes Intergovernmental Affairs Minister Stéphane Dion as saying that the uproar against appointing a separatist is "deplorable, but understandable." "Secession is very traumatic and you can't prevent people from thinking from time to time that their country is in danger." Dion notes, though, that Levine's opponents would be the first to become angry if a federalist were denied an equivalent job in Quebec. The page two story also recounts the uproar in the English language newspapers of Ottawa. Several readers, it says, find it odious to give such an important job to someone who has promoted separatism, and some fear that English will become a forbidden language.

In *Le Journal de Montréal* columnist Michel C. Auger, under the heading "Loyalty and intolerance," calls upon politicians to practise the virtues with which they claim to be inspired. The column recounts Levine's ethnicity and previous political involvement, mis-stating the date when he ran for office as 1989 rather than 1979:

> From nearly everywhere in the Ottawa area came a brutal and sometimes quite silly opposition, challenging the idea that a separatist would be capable of running a hospital in Ottawa. We won't give the list of stupidities which were expressed, it would be too long, but let's just say that an MPP[2] claimed that with Levine at the top, the newly amalgamated hospital would become "an institution devoted to the destruction of the country."
>
> The Ottawa newspapers followed this lead closely and asked

about the "loyalty" of Mr. Levine. They would like to acknowledge his abilities, but concerned themselves with whether he might be "anti-Canadian" or "disloyal to his country." A traitor, in other words?"

Since Mr. Levine does not want to speak of his political sympathies—as is his right in the strictest sense—and since he occupies a high level post for Quebec today and Ontario tomorrow, the Ottawa newspapers have pointed out that he could not have been named delegate general for Quebec without being sympathetic to the separatist cause. There is, in all this, a bit of a witch hunt that the late Senator McCarthy would not have disdained.

However, the Canadian Charter of Rights and Freedoms provides in Section 2 that each Canadian has the right to freedom of conscience and belief. There is no section making an exception for former PQ candidates.

That's why the Levine nomination is a subject about which we would like very much to hear from someone like Prime Minister Jean Chrétien, who likes to describe himself as the father of the Charter of Rights and Freedoms.

Is Mr. Chrétien, who doesn't fail to denounce the lack of tolerance, real or fictitious, of his sovereignist adversaries, ready to defend publicly Mr. Levine's freedom of belief? The true test of a defender of rights and freedoms, is readiness to make the defence even when it courts unpopularity.

Mr. Chrétien could begin by calling to account people in his party, such as M.P. Eugène Bellemarre who said that any separatist should be declared "persona non grata."

Or Stéphane Dion who says that the displays of intolerance were "unavoidable as long as we have the threat of separation."

One might well ask whether such people would be as understanding of intolerance if it happened in Quebec. If, for example, the people of Saguenay refused a hospital director because he was anglophone.

Hansard. The controversy has by now attracted national attention. It is worth comparing the media treatment with the following exchange, which takes place in the House of Commons. Questions from the BQ are brushed off with simple *ad hominem* ripostes, and a serious discussion of the issues is not achieved. The Liberals are ready for questions from the BQ, and manage to turn the tables on the questions about David Levine. The exchange takes place in French. The following is the English translation from Hansard.

Ms. Jocelyne Girard-Bujold (Jonquière, BQ): Mr. Speaker, my question is for the Deputy Prime Minister.

The government has a responsibility to ensure the enforcement of the Canadian Charter of Rights and Freedoms. Yesterday, the Minister of Intergovernmental Affairs once again added fuel to the fire by refusing to clearly condemn the demonstrations in opposition to David Levine's hiring to head the Ottawa Hospital.

By sanctioning this witch-hunt at Mr. Levine's expense, is the government not sending a message that the Canadian Charter of Rights and Freedoms does not apply to Quebec sovereignists or those under suspicion of being sovereignists?

Hon. Herb Gray (Deputy Prime Minister, Lib.): Mr. Speaker, I am pleased to see that the Bloc Québécois is now fully accepting the Canadian Constitution, including the Charter of Rights and Freedoms.

Ms. Jocelyne Girard-Bujold (Jonquière, BQ): Mr. Speaker, on the one side, we have the hon. member for Carleton-Gloucester also adding fuel to the fire by calling for Mr. Levine's dismissal because of his alleged political views. On the other, we have the hon. member for Ottawa-Vanier making far more respectful comments.

What exactly is the government position?

Hon. Don Boudria (Leader of the Government in the House of Commons, Lib.): Mr. Speaker, first of all, the federal government is not the one to hire or fire hospital directors, as you know. That is the role of the local board.

I too am very pleased to hear about the Bloc Québécois' respect for the Charter of Rights and Freedoms, particularly when, on September 29, 1994, the Deputy Premier of Quebec made a statement concerning a government employee to the effect that "A diplomat representing Quebec abroad who is unable to present the aspect of Quebec reality that is our path toward sovereignty is not qualified for this job."

A further exchange, this time in English, is also reported in Hansard, this time between the NDP and the Liberal government.

Mr. Dick Proctor (Palliser, NDP): Mr. Speaker, there is a witch hunt going on in the national capital. Some are calling for the resignation of David Levine, the new director of the Ottawa Hospital, because of his political beliefs.

All the Minister of Intergovernmental Affairs had to say about it was that it is deplorable, but understandable. Indeed, it violates the Charter of Rights and Freedoms.

Does the Deputy Prime Minister realize the damage caused to Canadian unity by the narrow-minded attitude of his colleague?

Hon Herb Gray (Deputy Prime Minister, Lib.): Mr. Speaker, the hiring of hospital directors does not concern the Canadian government in any way.

It is up to the individual to invoke the Charter of Rights and Freedoms if he feels that the policy of Ottawa hospitals infringes on his rights.

I think the Minister of Intergovernmental Affairs has done and continues to do a great job.

CFRA, **Lowell Green.** On May 15 Lowell Green devotes his talk show to the Levine affair. During the three-hour program points made in the newspapers are repeated, but Green's tone is aggressive and menacing. He expresses his hope that Patricia Bell, of CFRA, who is going to attend the Levine press conference that morning, will ask certain questions, which he then reads in a prosecutorial tone:

"1. Mr. Levine—Did you work at the Montfort Hospital during the early '70s, and Mr. Levine, what is your response to claims by co-workers that at that time you were a rabid separatist who refused to refer to Canada as anything other than a foreign nation? Has your opinion concerning Canada as a nation and its role *changed* since the 1970s?" Note that no names or evidence are provided for the allegation that he was a "rabid" separatist.[3] If there were concerns about Levine's freedom of expression, the tone of this questioning did not convey them. Green's questions echo the McCarthy era's famous "Are you or have you ever been a Communist?"

"2. Mr. Levine, have you offered jobs to anyone presently employed by the Quebec Government? Mr. Levine, have you offered jobs to any *senior* management staff from the Province of Quebec?" This is a particularly insidious question. He could hardly have offered any jobs because he had not yet taken up his position. But the fear-mongering suggestion is that Levine is some kind of fast operator.

"3. What is your position concerning an ongoing dispute between Ontario and the Province of Quebec over *payments* to both doctors and hospitals. For the past fourteen years or so Quebecers *refuse* to pay Ontario rates to Ontario doctors or Ontario hospitals." Figures similar to those provided by Dr. Charles Shaver were given.

"So I'd like to know, Mr. Levine, in a dispute of this nature between the government of the Province of Quebec and the Province of Ontario, if you are president of the Ontario Hospital, what will your position be—will you support the Ontario side in this? This is an example. And this is another side issue, folks, that we should deal with." Green then describes the $450 versus $745 fee differential.

"This has been going on for about fourteen years, folks, and we've put up with it. And you wonder why I, and a lot of people are asking questions about this. Mr. Levine, can we be guaranteed that you will support Ontario's position

and thus fly in the face of your friends in the Quebec government?" The implication of these questions is that Levine's position would be relevant to decision-making in such matters, which is a questionable assumption.

"One other question. Mr. Levine, did you or did you not pledge allegiance
to the separatist cause as recently as last year?" Lowell Green believes that the
PQ government requires all of its envoys to pledge allegiance to the cause of
Quebec sovereignty. "This is allegiance to a *cause*. In this case the cause of
breaking Canada apart. So Mr. Levine, did you or did you not pledge allegiance to the separatist cause as recently as last year?"

The tone of these questions is bullying and unreasonable. So what if Levine
pledged allegiance to the separatist cause? Separatism, one might point out, is
not an illegal option. The BQ is part of the Canadian loyal opposition, which
happens to seek a restructuring of the Canadian government to give additional
sovereign powers to Quebec. The idea that Levine would be disloyal to the
Ontario government is prejudicial. Were he to put his political allegiances ahead
of the duties of his job, that would be grounds for dismissal. Levine is being
treated as if he were guilty, and his failure to answer questions about his present
beliefs is seen as self-incriminating. What we are witnessing on this talk show
is contrary to the spirit of section 11(d) of the Charter of Rights and Freedoms,
namely, the presumption of innocence, whereby an accused person has the
right "to be presumed innocent until proven guilty according to law in a fair
and public hearing by an independent and impartial tribunal."

One caller, identified only as Mark, calls for tolerance. Mr. Green replies:
"This is not a matter of political belief—[but] a man who wishes to destroy this
country .... Demagoguery, my ass! ... Separatist ass-kissiness in Montreal.
Listen! This has got to stop!" He goes on to agitate against continuing to provide hospital services to Quebec patients. "We're getting screwed!"

Another caller identified as Gerry draws attention to one of many irritants
that have fuelled the opposition to Levine's appointment—Ontarians can't work
in Quebec. Taken literally and applied to all Ontarians, the statement is false,
but there have been well-publicized grievances about lack of reciprocity in the
construction industry.

During his press conference, which is broadcast live on Green's show.
Levine tells his audience about his love for health care work, saying that he
finds "nothing more interesting than the challenge to run and build the Ottawa
Hospital. I want this to become the best organization in Canada." He points out
that his previous hospital work was under both the PQ *and* the Liberals in Quebec: "I see myself as a bridge-builder." This is a "wonderful opportunity to
show the two founding nations can work together." He adds that there is no
intention to "impose penalties for being unilingual." Above all, he says, the
patient is to come first. Success depends upon motivating staff to offer the best
care and transparency and openness in the negotiations. "Team-building is key."
In the restructuring it would be important that "patients know where their doctors are." "The people come first," he says.

As for allegations about his separatism, he says he supports the "right of the people of Quebec to have a clear, open and democratic" choice. "I am a public servant" and "I have no political agenda," he says. "Wait and see," he counselled. If six months down the road, people don't like the results, they should do something.

Lowell Green follows up his coverage of the press conference with a question and a statement: "Is David Levine still a separatist? He's not going to answer this. Yet this is the only question that matters." He points out that when Levine was asked whether he had taken an oath of allegiance to a separate Quebec, he first said "No" and then qualified his answer to clarify that he was speaking specifically about his hospital job. As Green notes, he left open the question as to whether he had taken such an oath for his New York delegate general job. Once again, the viewpoint that Levine's political belief might be irrelevant in the new hospital job does not get a sympathetic hearing, if it is entertained at all.

Saturday, May 16

Ottawa Sun. This day marks a peak in coverage in the *Ottawa Sun.* Three full pages of news and columns are devoted to the previous day's press conference, together with an editorial entitled "Wrong," and a cartoon showing Levine entering his new office saying: "Actually ... I'd *prefer* my office to be in a *separate* building." This note of levity contrasts with the general tenor of the other writings.

Columnist Earl McRae has a full page instead of his usual column. His article, headed "The Separatist Shuffle," is accompanied by a photograph of CEO David Levine, and a smaller inset picture of Nicholas Patterson. Patterson was shown open-mouthed, hand cupped as if to amplify a shouting voice. The caption says he "complains about the use of French at the press conference."

McRae's opening lines are: "He's a separatist. No question about it." As evidence, he adduces Levine's answer to the question "Do you support philosophically the separation of Quebec from the rest of Canada." Levine's answer? "I support the aspirations of the people of Quebec to determine their own future in an open, democratic manner." Later, Levine repeated: "My previous answer was precise. I understand the views of Ottawa. I have no political agenda. But, I believe in the aspirations of the people of Quebec to determine their future in a democratic way." In McRae's view, this means: "I'm a separatist, and if my political beliefs result in the eventual secession of Quebec from confederation, so be it." Levine is quoted as saying, "I want to build bridges between the two communities; having to pass French tests is not my intention or that of the board," and "We do have to have services in both French and English, but it doesn't mean there won't be unilingual employees." To this McRae appends: "Doing what, sweeping floors?"

McRae describes Nicholas Patterson as "executive director of the Canadian Development Institute think tank," with no indication as to what the institute is about. A commotion developed, McRae writes, when Patterson shouted at Levine who had "lapsed" (McRae's word) into French: "Speak English. Or give us a translator. Most people here don't speak or understand French. This is supposed to be an English press conference." Patterson then refused a francophone woman's attempts to remove him from the room, according to McRae.

McRae quotes remarks Levine made directly to him and responds: "Levine's a separatist, I don't want a separatist running my hospital, he should be fired, the whole damn board should be fired. It's incompetent. Some people don't believe loyalty to your country matters. I do. Would the Americans allow a communist to be Secretary of State?"

McRae reacts in the same way to board chair Nick Mulder's statement that "The political, religious, or personal beliefs of the CEO, or of any of the hospital staff, are not relevant to the performance of his or her duties. At all times, the board must ensure that the best qualified person is appointed to any position." McRae replies, "I suppose, then, if Saddam Hussein had sent in his resume proving he has superior talent running a hospital, he'd be hired."

The *Sun's* editorial comments that while a public figure's religious beliefs are irrelevant, their political convictions are not. Levine was

> dead wrong ... when he insisted his political convictions were basically nobody's business. Well, they were everybody's business when he ran for election for the Parti Quebecois. And presumably they were an issue when he accepted a job as the separatist government's eyes, ears and mouth in New York City. And they're an issue today, here in a resolutely federalist region, no matter what he thinks to the contrary. Levine just doesn't seem to understand that residents of this region don't like separatists in their Parliament and don't want them running our hospitals ... Surely the board of trustees must now face up to their mistake and terminate Levine's appointment. Their job is to act in the best interests of the hospital and the public it serves. Better to correct a mistake now than live with its potentially disastrous consequences down the road.

The *Sun* prints what appears to be a verbatim transcript of the key sections of the conference on page 4, along with a story by Jacki Leroux, headed "The politics of confusion." It is about Levine's sidestepping of questions about his current political beliefs. Interestingly, she describes the press conference as being "before dozens of English and French reporters," which would seem to contradict Patterson's description of it as "an English press conference." Though written in the style of pure fact-reporting, the use of words like "while" and "but" subtly convey a judgement that Levine should have been more forthcoming:

While Levine, 50, said he supports "the aspirations of the people of Quebec" to "determine their own future," he refused to say—despite repeated drilling by reporters—whether he personally supports the separatist movement.

"I'm a Canadian citizen, I'm not a politician," he said. "I'm not here as a politician. I am a public servant, and I think people in Ottawa know what that means. I have no political agenda here," he said.

But Levine, who currently works as a PQ delegate promoting trade and investment in New York City, did add that he would like to see "bridges" built between the English and French in Canada, particularly in Ottawa.

Finally, the *Sun's* business editor, Stuart McCarthy, takes a stand on the Levine issue, with a column headed "Political beliefs infect hospital." He opens: "If David Levine has built any bridges between anglos and francophones, they must look like the Bridge over the River Kwai." Calling Levine's performance a "bob-and-weave show," McCarthy says Levine "has to go." He also questions Levine's support of the democratic will of Quebecers to separate:

> Was that the "democracy" that saw tens of thousands of ballots fraudulently discounted in majority English Quebec ridings during the last referendum?
>
> Or is it the "democratic" government that quashes the linguistic rights of minorities, blames "money and the ethnic vote" for losing the referendum and declares itself the champion of the "pure laine."

As McCarthy sees it, Levine's government is building one-way bridges to help Anglos, ethnics and anyone else opposed to the PQ separatist ways to leave Quebec. "Economic reality and consequences be damned."

Ottawa Citizen. The front page of the *Ottawa Citizen's* City section displays a four-column story about the reaction of area doctors to David Levine's appointment under the heading "MDs want secret vote on Levine," with the subhead "Appointment angers many doctors at Ottawa Hospital." The story is accompanied by a 7 inch by 5 inch photograph of Nick Mulder and a somewhat grim-faced David Levine.

According to this story, Jan Bormanis, president of the medical staff at the Civic site of the Hospital, spoke of "virtually unanimous support" at a meeting a few days earlier, which was attended by 200 doctors. "But some doctors say this does not accurately represent the views of the approximately 1,000 physicians in the hospital. 'I've talked to 40 doctors and I haven't hit on one yet that supports him. They are all outraged,' said Dr. Pete MacEwan, an anaesthetist, who attended the meeting." Robert Garnett, an anaesthetist at the Intensive

Care Unit of the Civic site, reportedly favours a secret ballot to better gauge physicians' opinions.

On the same page, in another story, Daniel Leblanc gives a run-down on the Levine coverage in the French media. He notes that Nicholas Patterson was given closeup coverage by RDI, the all-news French-language station, while he "was ranting about the fact that he couldn't understand parts of the press conference given in French." RDI also covered a woman, Barbara Lance, complaining about what she saw as excessive French coverage; in her view, since only 15 percent of the Ottawa Hospital's clientele speak French, only 15 percent of the press conference should have been in French. Leblanc adds, "The first half-hour of the press conference, however, was almost entirely in English. Mr. Levine's only words in French during his initial comments were to the effect that he was a unilingual anglophone until the age of 25." Leblanc also comments that much of what Levine said in French merely repeated what he had said in English.

Globe and Mail. The *Globe and Mail* gives the press conference page 4 placement, stressing David Levine's assertion that he has "no political agenda." The story, by Kevin Ward of Canadian Press, opens: "A hospital administrator under pressure to resign because of his separatist past defended his appointment yesterday by telling critics his politics aren't relevant to his work." It is on the whole sympathetic to Levine.

French Press. *Le Droit's* prominent banner headline on its front-page reports on Levine's previous day's press conference: "I am a bureaucrat" ("Je suis un fonctionnaire"). The story, by Isabelle Ducas, begins with a quotation affirming that Levine never dreamed of resigning, and that he was convinced he would be able to build bridges between the two communities. "I am not a politician," he is quoted as saying.

There is an inside story about MPP Garry Guzzo intensifying the pressure to rescind the Levine appointment. The story reminds readers that two years ago Guzzo proposed to the restructuring committee that Quebec workers should be laid off before Ontarians. Nicholas Patterson's interruption of Levine's French response to a question from *Le Droit* is noted.

In another story, Gisèle Lalonde, president of the Opération Constitution movement and the S.O.S. Montfort committee is quoted as saying that the same 20 percent of anglophones, bigots, are always the ones who intimidate politicians and sow fear in the general population.

Le Devoir carries a Canadian Press story by Kevin Ward about David Levine's protest that his political views would have no bearing on his job. The story notes that the *Citizen* and the *Sun* both suggested that Levine would likely be ineffective because of the controversy about his appointment.

Lise Bissonnette, publisher of *Le Devoir,* writes an editorial, "Repugnant," in which she speaks of the "hysterical outburst" ("crise d'hystérie") over the Levine appointment. In the eyes of the protesters, Levine was doubly wrong in being both a Quebecer and a separatist. She faults Intergovernmental Affairs Minister Stéphane Dion for describing the reaction as "deplorable but understandable." The root cause for the uproar was anxiety in the face of separatism, in Dion's view. This puts the fault on Levine, Ms. Bissonnette says; it's as if Levine's opinions started the problem.

Bissonnette believes that the reaction was caused by a level of nervous tension equal to that in the worst years of francophobia in the present and preceding centuries. The idea of sovereignty has existed for decades without inciting so much verbal violence, she notes. This recent flare-up was produced by a dual strategy designed by Stéphane Dion for implementation by the Canadian government. On the one hand, government manipulates public emotion so that the feeling of belonging to Canada, of flaunting it, of proclaiming it, and carrying out a noisy rally around the Canadian flag, is a *sine qua non* of citizenship. In the wave of passion that is generated, "separatists" become enemies rather than mere political opponents. On the other hand, the government adopts an elaborate theory which suggests that separation is illegal and that those who promote it are outlaws and traitors. Dion exploits this crisis. Look at how despised you will be, he is saying to Quebecers, if you persist in your bad thoughts. In Dion's strategy, it's all right to use threats and blackmail to combat separatism.

Sunday, May 17

Ottawa Sun. The *Ottawa Sun* continues to give the Levine affair extensive coverage. Half the Comments page is taken up with a cartoon showing a smug David Levine sitting at his office desk, saying "C'est la vie!" to the four microphones in front of him. The editor, Rick Gibbons, devotes a column to the issue, "Politics of convenience," in which he explores some of the reasons why Levine might have wanted to keep silent about his current political views. He notes that Levine would not have wanted to burn bridges behind him by renouncing separatism publicly, even if his views had changed.

Gibbons challenges the assumption that Levine's politics are his own business, and denies that such concern is McCarthyism: "Nobody's demanding that every bureaucrat, doctor or nurse swear an oath of allegiance or take an ideological means test." The point is rather that those who benefit from public political affiliations should also be prepared to accept disbenefits. The philosophy that "I have the right to publicly embrace any political option I want, even one that espouses the country's destruction, just don't hold me publicly accountable for it later on. My personal convictions are nobody's business, unless they get me a job in New York" just doesn't hold water. One cannot have it both ways. The public is right to say enough is enough, Gibbons concludes.

A news story on page five, "Docs divided on boss' politics," by Donna

Casey and Sarah Green, picks up material from the previous day's *Citizen* on the reaction of some physicians to the Levine appointment. The article speculates that the new head of the Ottawa Hospital "may have done more harm than good by skirting pointed questions about his political past." Disappointment on behalf of those who would have liked to have heard Levine renounce separatism is recorded. Brian Cayen, a biotechnologist at the General site of the hospital, is quoted: "All I wanted from him was a statement he believes in a united Canada." He fears for fund-raising efforts: "This is not anti-Quebec or anti-French. This is anti-separatist."

The story also questions the supposed widespread support for Levine among doctors. Peter MacEwan, anaesthetist at the Ottawa Hospital Civic site, feels the 200 pro-Levine votes the previous week were not a ringing endorsement of Levine. "I think the vote was completely meaningless," he is quoted as saying. He suggests that a mail-in survey of the hospital's 1,200 doctors would produce a more accurate picture. However, Dennis Pitt, head of the 2,000-member Ottawa Academy of Medicine, is reportedly confident that Levine would set aside his personal political views in the same way as do thousands of area residents who work as civil servants.

The *Sun* prints three letters against the Levine appointment. Bill Kielec congratulates Earl McRae for his May 14 column. Ray Grant argues that separatists can't have it both ways: "They cannot expect to work to break up Canada while at the same time accepting key positions in the country that they do not want to be a part of. Only in Canada do we have this absurd situation." Grant also attacks MP Mauril Bélanger for defending Levine. J.P. Redfern says that the Levine appointment should be nullified and that the board should be held accountable for "the offensive selection of an avowed enemy of a united Canada to preside over the primary health facility in this area."

Ottawa Citizen. While the *Ottawa Sun* is leading the charge against Levine and the board that hired him, the *Ottawa Citizen* provides counter-weight to these arguments. The first page of the City section gives prominent space to opinions favouring civil liberties and opposing any attempts to fire Levine or pressure him into resigning. The *Citizen* contacted me as a civil liberties activist and quotes me as comparing the attack on Levine to a McCarthy-type witch-hunt. "He is being attacked unfairly," I am quoted as saying. "You don't judge people on their racial, political or ethnic affiliation." Levine does not appear to be a "political animal," but "a civil servant first," I told the *Citizen*. The story further attributes to me the view that if Levine tried to use his new position to push his political agenda, he could be dismissed with just cause.

Other letter writers worry about a dangerous precedent. Errol Mendes, director of the University of Ottawa's human rights research and education centre, fears a slippery slope if agencies begin discriminating on political beliefs. He adds that he is a Canadian federalist but is deeply troubled by the reaction. Raj Anand, former chief commissioner of the Ontario Human Rights Commission, believes that firing Levine for being an alleged separatist would not be a breach of the Ontario human rights code. Human rights lawyer Emilio Binavince is quoted as seeing possible support for Levine in sections 2 and 15 of the Canadian Charter of Rights and Freedoms. Ottawa labour lawyer Steven Chaplin speculates that if Levine's appointment were terminated he would probably be compensated $165,000 or more.

Monday, May 18

Ottawa Citizen. The *Ottawa Citizen* gives the most prominent coverage to the Levine story with a front-page banner announcing that "Levine's hiring divides Ottawa." A poll commissioned by the *Citizen*, and conducted by COMPAS Inc. found that 52 percent of people surveyed the previous Friday and Saturday said that Levine "should be forced to resign," while 48 percent said he "should be allowed to stay on the job." A clear majority, 56 percent, lacked confidence in the committee that selected Levine. The poll also found that four out of five who thought that Levine should be fired held the view "strongly" or "very strongly." Only half of the 48 percent who supported Levine felt "strongly" or "very strongly." Sixty-four percent also agreed with the statement that "a separatist cannot be fair and objective dealing with Quebec." To COMPAS pollster Conrad Winn the overall implication is that "momentum is against [Levine]. The people who want his resignation feel very strongly about it. Those who want him to stay on feel very moderately about it."

The story also reports that MPP Garry Guzzo thinks that the poll underestimates the level of opposition to Levine's appointment. Guzzo is quoted as saying: "It's a 100-per-cent chance [the decision] will get reversed. It's a question of whether they do it this week or three weeks from now or six months from now .... We've put Mr. Levine in the position that he can't do his job .... He's in a lose-lose situation. The sooner the board realizes that the better."

Ottawa Sun. The *Ottawa Sun* also gives the Levine story front-page treatment, the angle being statements from Ottawa Hospital board members. "Levine hiring process flawed" proclaims inch-high type, with the subhead: "Hospital appointment outrage grows." Trustee Don Grant is quoted as saying that he is "not totally satisfied that [he] was getting a very good picture of what Levine's involvement with the PQ was." Those who defended the Levine appointment on the grounds that Levine's connection with separatism is something in the distant past appear less credible as more recent connections are stressed.

On page three, Earl McRae denounces the view that opposition to Levine amounts to McCarthyism, and implores his readers to show up at the next day's meeting of the Ottawa Hospital board to register their protests. He targets me for making the "bone-headed" charge that McCarthyism is involved in the opposition to Levine's appointment.

This is not about "McCarthyism," Mr. Randal Marlin, this is about the genuine, patriotic, wholly justified "*O Canada*-ism" that brave Canadians in two world wars fought and died for: A united Canada from sea to shining sea; not a Canada with a break-away country in its midst with its own foreign policy, its own military, its own adversarial political agenda. And if you and your Levine supporters can't grasp this, then do us a favor: Shut up, and go to bed.

My response to McRae's claims about McCarthyism appears in a *Citizen* essay published on May 25. McRae's column is worth further study, because it shows what a certain kind of thought constraint is all about. Everything is reduced to something simple that everyone can understand: If you love Canada, you must hate Levine's appointment. Those who disagree with you must be traitors to Canada.

What is missing is an important counter-argument. Some people believe that the failure to respect the entitlement of the separatist to a different vision of Canada is what may well hasten the departure of Quebec from Canada. Recall, for example, Paul Gaboury's remarks in *Le Droit* on May 5. It would not be difficult to respond to McRae in the same simplistic, militant tone he uses. In fact, some of the French columnists have used much the same kind of language to denounce the position exemplified in his column. This tone leads ultimately to Bosnian-style confrontations. In any event, it does little else than encourage the kind of shouting and boisterous behaviour witnessed on May 19 and widely broadcast across Canada.

The *Sun* also includes a detailed study of the procedures leading to Levine's appointment. The thirty-two members of the board are named; four of them are said to have abstained from voting. MPP Norm Sterling, the Government House Leader, is quoted as being "not happy with [Levine's] appointment" on the grounds that the job "has political overtones and overtures to it so therefore I think it's a poor choice." Garry Guzzo reportedly has received over 1,100 calls and close to 300 faxes protesting Levine's appointment. There was one letter in the *Sun* about Levine, calling the appointment a "drastic mistake," and seeking information about the board members.

French Media. *Le Journal de Montréal* columnist and well-known indépendantiste Pierre Bourgault writes that English Canada is going insane over the Levine affair. The newspapers have lit a fuse in calling for the resignation or immediate dismissal of "this monster who was readying himself to replace all the hospital employees by those nasty separatists, all while imposing French as the common language of work." He is right about the fuse, though reference to "this monster" would presumably reflect views of some letter-writers rather than editorial boards. Bourgault's other allegations are not directly attributable to the newspapers, though MPP Garry Guzzo's statements as quoted in the papers correspond to the image Bourgault presents.

Bourgault agrees with the argument made by Lise Bissonnette in her editorial, "Répugnant," but adds that the title is almost too weak. "I await the reaction of Jean Charest, as that of Jean Chrétien, as that of Mike Harris, as that of some citizens of English Canada who have not yet lost their heads," he wrote. "Catastrophe is still avoidable. For how long?" The reaction of Mike Harris was not long in coming, though perhaps it was not what Bourgault expected.

Tuesday, May 19, prior to meeting

Ottawa Citizen. The *Ottawa Citizen* devotes the top half of its City section to the Levine story, and the tone is somewhat negative. One story, headed "No politics, board warns Levine," reports a meeting on Friday May 15, between Nick Mulder, David Levine and *Citizen* editorial staff. The headline hints at tension between the hospital board and Levine. After all, those who have complete confidence in a new appointee don't need such a public "warning." The photo shows Levine's open mouth and half-closed raised hand. The caption is "The chairman of the hospital board Nick Mulder, right, explains he has advised David Levine, left, as he would any chief executive, 'You are not to go and use that job to promote your political or personal beliefs.' If he does, he will be fired."

On the top right of the page another story, "Hiring process 'flawed,'" reports the dissatisfaction of four members of the hospital board with the selection process. Board member Don Grant says that they abstained from voting for Levine and the selection committee failed in their obligation to present a short list of names to the board.

In contrast to the somewhat negative front page, the letters page of the City section has a very positive slant. A letter from Serge Menard of Verdun, Quebec, is full of praise for Levine and gets the headline "Levine is one of the best hospital administrators I've ever met." Menard, former chair of the verification committee at the Verdun Hospital which Levine headed, writes:

> I have found Mr. Levine to be one of the best administrators I have ever met .... Politics should not enter in judging the ability of a man to perform his duties. I am president of the Liberal Association of Verdun—St. Henri .... I am a convinced federalist, but I assure you politics were never a consideration of how Mr. Levine did his job .... [Y]ou should be grateful that the persons [who were] appointed to pick a man to run the Ottawa hospital, picked David Levine. As time will tell they could not have done better.

In a second letter, R. Scott Rowand of the Association of Canadian Teaching Hospitals, writing from Vancouver, says that the controversy over Levine is "perplexing":

Mr. Levine is respected across Canada as a competent, committed and highly professional health care executive. He possesses the skills, attributes, and knowledge necessary to provide the leadership required by the Ottawa Hospital for the mammoth task set by the Health Service Restructuring Commission. Mr. Levine should be welcomed by the citizens of Ottawa and offered all the support he will need.

Frank Laverty writes to urge Ottawa-Carleton residents and corporations to "cancel their donations to the Ontario political parties until the ugly mess in our health care is settled to the satisfaction of the public."

Ottawan Susan Menzies, President of the Heart Institute Foundation, writes that the University of Ottawa Heart Institute was administered differently from the Ottawa Hospital: "We have been, and continue to be, governed by our own board of directors with a separate charitable foundation and a research corporation."

Janice Treciokas of Ottawa humorously asks how could a separatist, philosophically, countenance amalgamation?

Raymond Hurtubise of Ottawa detects more than fear against separatism in the opposition to Levine; he sees an anti-French attitude. Could Levine's statement that he intends to keep the former General Hospital a bilingual institution "be what's really behind all those letters and calls from mostly English-speaking people?" he asks. Hurtubise adds: "I also detect a hatred against the French-speaking people—most of the complaints I read would appear to come from people with feelings similar to the Association *(sic)* for the Preservation of English in Canada, or Union Jack advocates or any other racist sympathisers." His only concern was that the most competent person be hired.

Roger Cain of Ottawa adopts a mocking tone regarding the many separatists or former separatists working in Ottawa, whose politics he had previously ignored: "I thought that Canada was a free country and that employment was independent of one's politics. However, continued reading of the current demagoguery has shown me the error of my ways." He now realizes that the "excellent, competent work" performed by a separatist he knew was "probably just a cover until they could participate in the destruction of everything that is near and dear to us all." These people, he says with heavy irony, "must be considered guilty until proven innocent. Immediate removal from positions and incarceration until proven innocent. We must act, before it is too late."

Ottawa Sun. *The Ottawa Sun* gives Levine front-page attention with a four-line, one-inch typeface headline: "Hospital board on hiring hot seat." Inside, a story by Donna Casey is bannered "Hospital showdown looms." The subhead notes, correctly as it turned out, "Sparks set to fly as board faces public's wrath on Levine issue." The story portrays Barbara Ramsay, a community representative on the hospital board, as dissatisfied with the selection procedure:

"Many people feel the Levine deal was a done deal before the board had a chance to discuss it. I have a problem with that."

Peter Clark, former regional chair and a member of the board strongly denounces the media: "Frankly I think the people who have been promoting this divisiveness—i.e. the media—are doing more to divide Canada than what's ever been done in my history."

A sidebar story airs the views of board member Robert Leitch alongside a 5 inch by 6 inch photo of him outside the General site. If Levine were forced to resign or were fired, the job of CEO would be tainted, in Leitch's view; it would be "real trouble selecting anyone for the new one." The job was not supposed to be political but it has become so, he said.

An editorial, "Listen," says it has become apparent that the hospital board is becoming "as divided as the public it serves," arguing that the board would have to revisit the hiring and rescind it, "even if it means the hospital will be on the hook for hundreds of thousands of dollars in penalties." The mistake was made by a rookie board, it said, and the lesson should be that "even an unelected board of directors is still accountable for its decisions."

The *Sun* also devotes a full page of letters to the Levine controversy, along with a 6 inch by 4 inch reprinting of the "C'est la vie" cartoon. An influential letter of the day, written by Andrew Caddell of Geneva, Switzerland, faults Levine for saying no more about his PQ past than he did of his candidacy in the D'Arcy McGee riding in 1979. He draws attention to Levine's close friendship with Bernard Landry who is "hardly a role model of discretion and neutrality." To have held a post as delegate general in New York for the PQ government, Levine would have had to sign a commitment to promote the separatist option, Caddell claims. He should resign because "misleading the public and the board of trustees on as basic an issue as his professional past and political philosophy is not a good way to develop public trust in such an important institution."

The first letter, from François LeMay of Vanier, suggests that, by parallel reasoning, federalists working in Quebec should be fired. The *Sun*'s comment is: "No deal—we don't put people who want to keep the country together in the same boat as someone who wants to tear it apart."

Comparisons to other threats to freedom of belief are made by Bob McLarty, who notes that people are already sensitive about the pro-choice or gay rights views of a potential administrator and that he deplores adding separatism to the list.

Denis M. Lynch charges Levine with assuming that the well-being of a hospital is independent of the well-being of the community it serves, and that the well-being of the capital is independent of the well-being of the country. No basis for his claim is given. The *Sun* appends the remark: "With the way he's skating around the issue, it's a little difficult to figure out what he thinks at all … and he doesn't seem to want us to know."

M. Henrie writes to say that bigotry is flourishing and that Levine attackers are pursuing contradictory goals: "On the one hand, indulging in Quebec bashing, and on the other, wanting it to stay in confederation." The *Sun* replies: "Insofar as Levine isn't a French Quebecer, we have trouble following your logic."

Pat Rowley remarks on the stupidity of the "Levine-Mulder farce" and blames Ottawa generally. The *Sun* conceded, "It's not our brightest moment."

Frank Simek of Braeside attacks Nick Mulder for equating Levine's political beliefs to affiliation with a religion or the Reform Party. Adopting a philosophy that calls for the breakup of Canada is different, Simek claims. "Whether Levine stays or not, Mulder must go," he wrote.

Jack MacLean of Gloucester lightly comments that he would not, as an engineer, have much faith in a bridge designed by David Levine: the bridges Levine wanted to build were between a separatist party and the anglophones, but the former want to destroy Canada.

Jack MacKinnon, President of the Civil Liberties Association of the National Capital Region, proposes that Levine would likely be competent; that his separatist background would probably not affect his performance; that he could be released with cause if it did; that to renege on his contract would probably be more damaging to Canadian unity than keeping him; and that donors withholding funds were doing so unreasonably.

John Courtenay writes to congratulate Earl McRae and the *Sun* for their efforts to have the "disgraceful" appointment cancelled.

W.J. Zlepnig protests the hiring, suggesting that the methods and action of separatism are tantamount to "treason": it would be wrong to accept one of their followers cloaked "in a pin-stripe suit to administer two of our Canadian hospitals."

J. Stevens complains that "English Canadians are frequently denied hiring or promotion for language reasons, although they are the best qualified for the job."

French Media. Both *Le Devoir* and *Le Droit* report from the Canadian Press that the Canadian Jewish Congress of the Quebec region deplores the negative reactions to David Levine's appointment. Dorothy Zalcman Howard, president of the organization, says in a communiqué: "Freedom of opinion and conscience are the basis of our democratic life. It is truly regrettable that certain individuals currently choose to deny these fundamental principles and are prepared to condemn a very distinguished administrator for having wrong opinions." *Le Droit* also carries a cartoon of the blindfolded figure of justice with hands bound by tubing from two different blood supplies.

A letter from D. Ménard of Ottawa asks whether Ontario foresees workers from Quebec having to take an oath as a test of loyalty. He also asks:

> Does the Ontario employer have the right to inquire into the political convictions of job applicants, and to make them a criterion of selec-

tion that is more important than the ability to do the job well? Is it really the political affiliations of David Levine that are at the origin of this uproar or is it rather the fact that he intends to offer services as much in French as English?

Mr. Ménard hopes that French services will not be compromised by the political tempest. He also notes that, while the Ontario health minister was asking the Ottawa Hospital to "reconsider" its hiring, the House of Commons was taken up with a private member's bill, supported by five political parties, to recognize Louis Riel as a Father of Confederation—he who had been hanged as a traitor.

On radio, Lowell Green urges his listeners to attend the meeting scheduled for that night. If there isn't a large turnout, he says, this will be taken as approval of the hiring: "The board has got to understand that the vast majority of this community opposes this." He informs his listeners that the meeting has a new location in the amphitheatre of the Civic hospital site. Green conducts his own opinion poll, asking whether Levine should be fired or retained. By his own count, the numbers were forty-three in favour of firing him and five in favour of retaining him. One caller, "Roger from Gatineau," says that Green's show polarizes people and gets them "frenzied up": "It seems you bring out the worst on this show," he said. Green followed this with the remark that Levine had been done out of a job in Montreal by "rabid nationalists." The opposition to Levine was not anti-French, Green said, but anti-separatist.

The overall coverage in the media set the stage for public opinion and reaction. Although the *Citizen* had begun printing some pro-Levine considerations, it did not do so early enough to significantly affect its general anti-Levine stance. The *Sun* and CFRA Radio were militantly supporting the anti-Levine side. In light of this, the performance of the crowd later that evening was more or less to be expected.

Notes

1. It should be noted that Dale Hibbard's letter itself involves name-calling (Eugène Bellemare and Garry Guzzo are called "nincompoops" who "simple-mindedly" decried the appointment of David Levine, and who made use of "asinine logic"), and so tends to encourage extreme language in reply.
2. The reference was presumably to MPP Garry Guzzo.
3. It is also worth noting that the word "rabid" means "furious, raging" or "madly violent in nature or behaviour" (Oxford English Dictionary).

CHAPTER THREE

THE PUBLIC MEETING, MAY 19, AND REACTIONS

The pinnacle of the David Levine affair, as a media event, was the May 19 meeting at the Civic hospital site, where Ottawa Hospital board members faced the hostile public for the first time. Those who were anticipating and dreading an unproductive slanging match stayed away unless motivated by a sense of public duty. The audience included a high proportion of retirees. Some decorated Second World War veterans marshalled patriotic displays against Levine. Pro-Levine speeches were shouted down. Television images of the boisterous meeting reached television sets across Canada, as the story was catapulted onto the national stage. According to André Picard's May 21 *Globe and Mail* article, it was "the week's hottest political story." The French language media contrasted the behaviour of this crowd with the anti-separatist "Quebec we love you" federalist rally in Montreal prior to the October 1995 referendum.

The scene was revolting to many who value civilized discourse. Some who had not supported Levine were nonetheless appalled at the manifestation of hostility, creating a watershed in public opinion and eroding some anti-Levine support. Backlash eventually became evident in letters to the newspapers. In the build-up to the meeting, however, some politicians felt it important to support the public mood with personal letters or telephone calls.

On the same day, Ottawa Mayor Jim Watson said that Levine should resign so as not to impede fundraising efforts. On the following day, Ontario Premier Mike Harris let his support for the anti-Levine people be known, producing page one headlines on May 21 and airing his views on a widely reported Toronto radio talk show. The *Citizen* quoted him: "Given that [separatist] background, and if that's what he still believes in, he wouldn't have been our first choice. Surely there is administrative capability within Ontario, or at least a Canadian or even a non-Canadian who believes in Canada and keeping Canada together." The French translation in *Le Devoir* read: "Given his past and what he still believes, he would not have been our first choice. I am sure there are capable administrators in Ontario ...."

But statements from politicians dissociating themselves from the anti-Levine mentality, Prime Minister Jean Chrétien among others, were also forthcoming. It was still not clear whether the board would stand firm, but on May

21 when it made public its unanimous decision to do so (with 28 members present out of 32), the real turnaround began. We began to see, in the *Citizen,* more stories emphasizing Levine's positive attributes. At least one columnist, Susan Riley, backtracked from her previous position. Others, notably Earl McRae, hardly budged. But, except for a small minority who boycotted the businesses of board members as late as July 1998, the overall tenor became one of reluctant acquiescence.

Tracking shifts in public opinion, as reflected in the media, requires careful attention to dates and times. Letters to the editor are particularly problematic because the date of publication often bears little relation to the date of submission. Letters can be saved and later grouped together to tell a story or fit well with an editorial. Letter writers' ideas can be used in news stories, so that the letter appears to reinforce or complement what the newspaper has said, rather than inspiring it. Letters are often edited, usually to lend clarity and avoid repetition, and sometimes to suppress things the editor would prefer not to see in print. As a result, it becomes difficult to keep a clear focus on the unfolding of ideas and events in the media.

For easy reference, I have highlighted events of and following the May 19 meeting:

May 19: The meeting, with its attention-capturing television images of crowd hysteria, hatred, and intolerance.

May 20: The coverage of the meeting in the print media, with prominent front-page treatment; Ontario Premier Mike Harris's statement; a statement by Intergovernmental Affairs Minister Stéphane Dion; a statement by Liberal Opposition Leader Dalton McGuinty; Prime Minister Jean Chrétien speaks in Rome.

May 21: Prominent reports on the previous day's statements by politicians; announcement by the Ottawa Hospital board reconfirming the Levine appointment but apologizing for having aroused passionate feelings it had not anticipated; Quebec Premier Lucien Bouchard, in Chicago, reacts to Premier Harris's statements; the Quebec National Assembly unanimously adopts a motion denouncing intolerance shown towards David Levine.

May 22: Prominent report of Bouchard's comments and of the decision in Quebec; Prime Minister Chrétien comments again from Italy on the affair.

May 23: Reports on Chrétien's remarks.

Editorials and commentary were at their height in the latter part of the week, continuing into the next week. The position espoused by the *Ottawa*

Sun, the *Ottawa Citizen* and CFRA seemed parochial and isolated compared with the media in the rest of the country, French or English.

In the following review, some letters will be greatly summarized and others only mentioned; no offence is meant to letter writers who get short shrift. Many points are repeated, especially from one newspaper to the next.

Wednesday, May 20

This was the first opportunity for the print media to cover the previous night's explosive meeting. Most main stories comment upon the uproar and expressions of intolerance, but also the very strong support for the anti-Levine, anti-board position. What follows are accounts from various newspapers and the Canadian Public Affairs Channel videotape of the proceedings, as well as from interviews with some of those present.

Le Droit. *Le Droit* has a front-page headline in inch-high type: "Levine à la porte!" ("Out with Levine!"). A 7 inch by 5 inch photograph shows a young man, identified as Joe Lemaire, carrying a picture of Levine with an "X" marked across it and the words "NO SEPERATISTS" *(sic)*. The subhead summarizes the meeting: "The opposition to the Levine hiring as head of the Ottawa Hospital reached a paroxysm yesterday evening, when an angry crowd demonstrated noisily in front of the 32 members of the new hospital board."

"For three hours," writes Isabelle Ducas,

> the board listened to questions from about fifty people, mostly people who described themselves as federalists outraged to see a "separatist," a "traitor who wants to destroy the country," as the head of their hospital. Several asked for the resignation of David Levine and of the whole board, encouraged by the cries of the crowd, who repeated in chorus "Resign! Resign!" or who chanted "Shame on you!"

Ducas's story noted that even Mauril Bélanger, Ottawa-Vanier MPP, was greeted with the shout "separatist" when he came to the microphone to explain that it would be discriminatory to dismiss anyone because of their political beliefs, and that separatists also had rights. It was Bélanger, she observed, who had organized the huge pro-federalist rally in Montreal on October 27, 1995, the eve of the referendum.

Ducas noted that only one person, Jacques Schayburt, spoke in French, congratulating the board for its courage until the crowd yelled at him to speak English. Brenda Cooper, who described herself as being of white, Anglo-Saxon, Protestant origin, expressed shame and anger at the behaviour of the crowd. She said that her father and grandfather, who fought for democracy, must be turning in their graves to see this bullying.

Le Droit printed two more stories, with photographs, on page four. In one of them, Denis Gratton noted the contrast between MP Mauril Bélanger and MP Eugène Bellemare. The latter had said a week earlier that Levine should not have been nominated to the position in view of his 1979 candidacy for the separatist party. Bélanger by contrast said that "as long as [Levine] agrees to leave his political opinions out of it, he is an ideal candidate for the job. And Levine has clearly accepted that condition." The picture shows a concerned and worried Bélanger being hectored by angry participants at the meeting.

Adjacent to the Gratton article is Charles Thériault's report on the views of Jim Durrell and Jacqueline Holzman. Both were former Ottawa mayors active in the organization called Patients First, which lobbied for maintaining most services at the Civic site. Thériault notes that Durrell is somewhat ambivalent and quotes him: "If [Levine] feels that he has the confidence of the board the doctors and the public, then he should continue. If not, he should leave."

Two letters are published. One is by Jack MacKinnon, a translation of what appears in English in the *Sun*. The other is by Johannes Martin Godbout of Gatineau, who says that Levine's freedom of belief is not being respected, and that there is growing evidence that opposition to Levine stems from his mandate to assure equal service in French and English alike. Though not much spoken about, Levine's Jewishness seems not to have helped him, Godbout thought.

Montreal French Media. *La Presse* quotes at the top of its front page "Levine est un traître." Vincent Marissal says that the spite and intolerance of the David Levine "trial" in the newspapers has led the national unity debate to one of its darkest hours. "About 500 people, the great majority over 60, spent more than three hours telling—yelling would be a more appropriate word—the board members of the Ottawa megahospital that they did not want a separatist in their institutions." The story has special praise for the courage of MP Mauril Bélanger and discusses some of the background to the meeting.

Le Journal de Montréal's Canadian Press story on page 22 is headed "Acute crisis of discrimination in Ottawa" and appears to be a re-write of *Le Droit's* story.

Ottawa Citizen. Coverage of the Levine affair is very extensive, several pages in all. The *Citizen* devotes a foot square of space on its front page to two pictures of the meeting, one of former Ottawa mayor Marion Dewar, and another of a woman carrying a "no seperatists'" *(sic)* placard. The headline in one-inch type reads "The battle over David Levine," and the subhead, "Foes, defenders of new hospital CEO square off in emotional debate over administrator's separatist past."

The lead paragraph of the story, jointly written by Pat Bell, Mark Gollom and Dawn Walton, takes a neutral stance, playing up the opposed factions:

"Former Ottawa mayor Marion Dewar and Second World War veteran Daniel O'Dwyer represented the two major emotions last night as close to 500 people gathered to air their views over the appointment of David Levine as head of the newly amalgamated Ottawa Hospital."

The next two paragraphs describe the bullying crowd. When Dewar said, "The candidate appears to have fulfilled the requirements for the appointment," the audience responded with a chorus of roars of "Out, out, out," the story said. When she continued, "The controversy has concentrated on his past political activity," the crowd drowned her out with more shouting.

The story reported that the amphitheatre of the Civic site of the hospital was filled half an hour before the scheduled meeting with the board. "War veteran Mr. O'Dwyer, wearing his uniform and medals, received a standing ovation even before he spoke." He said: "Four famous regiments from Quebec fought in the war, but [Levine] has tried to destroy what I fought and bled for. You members of the board are no better than him. I hope you don't wear a poppy on the 11th of November."

The crowd sang *O Canada* before the meeting began, the story says, and repeated the anthem again at the end of the meeting at 9 p.m. More than 35 people spoke into the microphones, two-thirds adamant that Levine not take up the appointment. "Over and over, people chanted 'resign! resign!' and 'Nick Mulder must go.'"

Wade Wallace, director of a unity group called Solidarité Outaouais Solidarity, is quoted as saying, "Mr. Levine should be fired whatever the cost. It's time these people paid the cost for their political choice. Our unity group can't celebrate Canada Day in Hull. We don't want anti-Canadians in our hospitals."

The *Ottawa Citizen* also gives the Levine controversy and the previous night's meeting considerable space (10 inches by 11 inches) on the front page of its City section. At the top is a picture of two men carrying signs that say "Levine go home" and "Fire Levine and the board."

The headline raises a different matter: "Mayor urges Levine to quit." The lead paragraph reads "The head of the new amalgamated hospital should 'do the honourable thing and resign' for the good of the institution, Ottawa Mayor Jim Watson said yesterday." Watson's main concern seems to be that Levine's appointment would hurt fundraising efforts.

The story also reports that Gloucester Mayor Claudette Cain questioned whether Levine, given his political affiliations, could keep his political beliefs separate from his role as the head of a public institution. "His mandate is to run the hospital [but] human nature says he has beliefs that want to destroy our country and somehow, somewhere it infiltrates into your persona."

A useful list of biographies of the thirty-two members of the hospital board of directors is provided inside the City section. There is a full page of letters, and a sympathetic column by Randall Denley, "Let Levine get on with his job," which resulted from a meeting with David Levine. "It's a stretch to think

Levine's involvement with the Parti Québécois will affect his job performance at the hospital. It's rather unlikely that Levine would do anything that would be seen as sympathetic to the PQ," Denley writes.

The letters page balances both unfavourable and favourable opinions on the Levine affair. The one-inch headline also does not take sides: "Levine: should he go—or stay?"

Letters by Ottawans Norman Levine, Robert Lemieux and Ann Young draw parallels with McCarthyism. In his prominently placed letter, Levine (no relation) directs strong criticism against the *Citizen's* coverage:

> David Levine has been vilified and targeted by a media attack, led by the *Citizen*, to the immense shame of that once respected newspaper. That the *Citizen* would conduct a "poll," call it news, and make it the headline on May 18, thus essentially manufacturing the very news that it is purporting to report, would be merely outrageously bad journalism, were it not actually dangerous and destructive to the unity of our country.

Hubert Gratton of Ottawa praises the courage of the hospital board in standing by its principles, and he announces that he is reaching for his cheque-book in support.[1] Melissa Coleman of Ottawa defends Levine's Charter freedoms and argues that the best health care should be the main concern, not politics. Dominique Joly of Vanier says that for the sake of this country's unity it would be better to "hold out your hands to Quebecers" and not "spit in their face."

Laurence C.N. Burgess of Nepean and Brian Gifford of Ottawa both think that the best qualified person should be offered the job. Burgess even sees Levine as "a gift from God—a fluently bilingual anglophone Jew with impeccable credentials who will administer well in a difficult position."

Among the eight letters opposed, E. Kinsella of Ottawa says that he changed his favourable outlook on the appointment after learning about the shortfall in medical fees from Quebec to the Ontario system, and about possible problems regarding hiring and firing of anglophone workers. A further concern was Levine's apparent lack of forthrightness in answering questions about his separatist connections.

Tonia Kelly of Manotick says that Levine must go, even though the payout would likely be obscene, and that the board should be drastically reduced in size. Margaret Labarge of Ottawa argues that the hospital board has shown itself to be "out of touch with the community whose health care they are expected to manage." If they did not expect a major reaction to the appointment of a current official of the PQ government to the Ontario Hospital administration "they have shown a lack of foresight and a misunderstanding of the local community." The board's competence "has been seriously undermined by this mistaken judgement." She does not, however, call specifically for any resignations.

Peter Janeck thinks that Levine is of questionable trustworthiness, giving as evidence a report that Levine told Americans that "their businesses would in no way be bothered or affected by separation." "Only a fool or a liar could say that," Janeck claimed.

Peter A. Ludwig of Nepean scornfully challenges the supposition that Levine was simply a public servant, given the prominent political names with which he has been associated. F. Gary James, Geoffrey Wastenays, and Bob Allen also have letters critical of the board and Levine's appointment.

Ottawa Sun. The *Ottawa Sun's* front-page, two-line headline in one-inch type screams at the reader: "Bitter crowd hammers board." The *Sun* is in the middle of its sequence of five-day front-page coverage of the topic, and has clearly taken over from the *Citizen* the role of chief cheerleader for the forces opposing Levine and the board. The subhead on the front page reads: "Hundreds demand 'separatist' Levine, hospital trustees resign." An elderly man and a woman are photographed, mouths wide open, fists raised and anger in their faces. The man holds miniature Canadian flags in his left hand. Second World War veteran Frank Laverty is quoted: "First of all, admit your damn error. Second of all correct it. I'm very annoyed .... The board should resign."

Earl McRae's column covers the meeting like a sports event:

> And, they sang *O Canada*, over and over in deafening voice, and they chanted over and over: "Mulder Must Go!" and "Get Rid Of Levine!" and "Resign! Resign! Resign!"
>
> One older man, his blazer bedecked with medals, stood up and shouted that 140,000 Canadian soldiers died for Canada, and when a Levine supporter yelled at him, "What side are you on?" he stormed over to him, stuck his medals in his face, and spat: "Freedom—what side are *you* on?"
>
> The crowd roared its approval.

By the tone of his report, McRae seems to approve of this kind of conduct. These people were, to him, representing "real life" as distinct from "fairy-land." It was a "call to arms" to show the "forces of separatism they will not be seduced into submission."

Two full pages are taken up inside the *Sun*. The top story by Sarah Green headed "Tempers flare over CEO hiring," recounts the emotionalism of the meeting, contributions by Second World War veterans and support for Levine by MP Mauril Bélanger and Marion Dewar. The story also quotes lawyer Paul Webber as saying that the board should stand by its decision. He denounced the mob mentality of the crowd and urged them to respect his freedom of speech: "This is McCarthyism, plain and simple." Pictures of Marion Dewar, Nick Mulder, two demonstrators and police expelling Bob Guzzo, identified as a cousin of MPP Garry Guzzo, are shown.

On the Comment page, the *Sun* has a cartoon of Levine at his desk saying "Go home ... Drink plenty of fluids ... and take a Prozac!" By contrast, the *Sun* publishes Roger Davidson's strongly critical letter against Earl McRae's May 18 column. There was, Davidson writes, a "definite smell of McCarthyism." He does not claim to be knowledgeable about Levine's qualifications. "I do, however, take strong exception to being told to 'shut up and go to bed' if I don't agree with Mr. McRae's jingoistic ramblings," he writes. He sees McRae's writings as causing more harm to Canadian unity than "anything Mr. Levine could ever do in his position."

Toronto Newspapers. The *Financial Post* column by Ottawa lawyer Arthur Drache, a specialist in charities, comments on the power of the people to make their voices heard "in a tangible fashion" by threatening to withhold gifts and bequests. The new hospital board apparently concluded that Levine's political beliefs were irrelevant, but "They should have thought again," he writes.

The *Toronto Star* gives the meeting about 26 column-inches of coverage in a story headed "Angry crowd demands firing of separatist hospital official." The report by Mark Bourrie says:

> Most of those in the crowd were seniors who applauded Tara Barclay when she said, "It is my understanding that Mr. Levine got his amalgamation expertise by closing English hospitals in Quebec and removing English language signage in the French hospitals, thereby complying with Quebec's Bill 101, a bill that abuses the English-speaking citizens of Quebec. Is Ontario to become an extension of Quebec, where English rights are trampled upon? Because of this, Mr. Levine should resign and the board should do likewise."

The *Globe and Mail* editorial, "Separating politics and business," comes down very strongly in favour of tolerance and of judging David Levine on his skills as a hospital administrator rather than on his politics. It questions the fairness of those who fear increased use of French:

> People have wondered aloud whether Mr. Levine would promote francophones and ignore anglophones. That speaks volumes about where the antipathy to him lies; unless, of course, these same people were similarly up in arms a couple of years ago about the announced closing of Ottawa's only French-language hospital, the Montfort, and fretting about the implications of that decision. Judging from the sound and fury of this controversy, in fact, it is Mr. Levine's critics, not Mr. Levine, who are having trouble keeping politics in perspective.

THURSDAY, MAY 21

The reaction against the mob mentality of Tuesday's meeting begins to be felt strongly in the media. Prime Minister Jean Chrétien reportedly spoke out the day before in Rome against firing Levine because of his PQ connections. The Quebec Legislature passes a motion denouncing the intolerance shown against David Levine and "reiterating the importance of respecting, in our democratic society, the fundamental principle which is freedom of opinion." The French newspapers react indignantly to comments by Ontario Premier Mike Harris that sympathized with the noisy crowd at Tuesday night's meeting. The David Levine affair has now become firmly entrenched as a national issue.

Le Devoir. Le Devoir gives a prominent headline in half-inch type on its front page: "Harris adds fuel to the fire." The story by Manon Cornellier and Mario Cloutier is highly critical of Harris's statement the previous day that he was "on the side of" those who thought that taxpayers' money should not be used to hire a "separatist." Apparently had he a choice, he would prefer hiring a foreigner who was a federalist: "Given his past and what he still believes, he would not have been our first choice. I am sure there are competent administrators in Ontario or that there is at least a Canadian or even a non-Canadian who believes in Canada and in a united Canada," was what Le Devoir attributed to Harris.[2] It's also worth mentioning that the word "Anglophonies" appears next to the Levine story. The word heads an article about Alliance Quebec, but it resonates with the Levine story.

An inside cartoon shows an angry mob carrying "Down with Levine" signs and a British bulldog holding a maple leaf flag in its teeth. A foaming, openmouthed, medal-toting veteran is shaking a finger and holding a flag in the other hand. A smiling Sheila Copps says, in front of the Ottawa Hospital, "It's nice to see how my flags are used."[3]

A story by Pierre O'Neill focuses on the views of Intergovernmental Affairs Minister Stéphane Dion, who is quoted as describing the conduct of the crowd at Tuesday's meeting as "inexcusable"; it's understandable, but to explain something is not to excuse it, he said. Dion reportedly said that he has a number of *indépendantiste* friends and that there was never any question in his mind of excluding them because of their political convictions. "This is the kind of intolerance which must be put to an end," he said. "Mr. Levine is the best candidate, so he should manage the hospital .... The history of Canada is not made by excluding people, but through dialogue."

A story by Isabelle Paré goes into David Levine's background, noting how he came to the assistance of Bernard Landry in the ministry of economic development and how he has since maintained ties with Landry. But his main reputation was made in the health system, where he gained a reputation as a knowledgeable and innovative administrator. Heading the Notre-Dame Hospital in 1992, he lost this position during the amalgamation with two other hospitals when Quebec opted for a "neutral candidate," one not affiliated with any of the three hospitals, according to this report.

Winnipeg Free Press. A Canadian Press story by Janice Tibbetts is published in the *Winnipeg Free Press* (and other newspapers) on page 11, under the prominent head, "Hospital hiring sparks unity battle." The leading paragraphs state:

> Ottawa—A dispute over hiring a former Parti Quebecois candidate to head an Ottawa hospital exploded into a national unity battle yesterday, pitting separatists against federalists as David Levine waited to hear whether he would lose his job.
> Politicians from Prime Minister Jean Chretien in Rome to Quebec Premier Lucien Bouchard in Chicago jumped into the debate over whether Levine's sovereigntist past makes him the right choice to run Ottawa Hospital, the city's newly amalgamated mega-hospital.[4]

The story is 16 column inches and recounts a lot of the history, including the Ottawa newspapers' call for Levine's resignation. It also quotes Bloc Québécois leader Gilles Duceppe as saying that the outcry against Levine is "a very bad signal for Canada. It means Canada is no longer a tolerant society," and Quebec Premier Lucien Bouchard as saying, "I am as surprised as many people to see this outburst of intolerance. I count on the good sense and democratic values of our fellow citizens in Ottawa to lower the tone [i.e., decibels rather than taste] and recognize what counts in all of this is competence."

Le Journal de Montréal. *Le Journal de Montréal* gives extensive treatment to the story, with two facing pages devoted to the Levine reaction, under a general rubric, "The Anti-Levine Movement." The left-hand headline reads: "David Levine … a competent hospital administrator, ignored by Quebec and rejected in Ottawa!" Michelle Coude-Lord emphasizes Levine's competence and says that Quebec had handed "one of its most competent administrators to Ontario." Though Levine wanted badly to continue with his main area of competence, "too much is too much. The storm which he is currently weathering in Ottawa has profoundly hurt the competent administrator and the man he is."

On the facing page a story by Laurent Soumis describes Ontario Premier Mike Harris's intervention as "oil on fire" and quotes Quebec vice-premier Bernard Landry's response: "To say that a foreigner is preferable to a Quebecer because of his political opinions is not what I call calming the situation." Landry also called on Stéphane Dion to denounce the affair in unequivocal terms to "stop the drift of public opinion" in English Canada.

A third story, also by Laurent Soumis, analyses Earl McRae's call to arms in the *Ottawa Sun,* mentions Arthur Drache's *Financial Post* article and summarizes the *Globe and Mail* editorial of the previous day. The *Ottawa Citizen's* views are also summarized in an account of Randall Denley's column.

A column by Franco Nuovo, headed "The trial," characterizes the violent opposition to Levine as "disguised racist expression in the form of repression and backed up by the hypocrisy of politicians. How has Canada fallen so low?"

Nuovo says that Levine was rejected, not because he is Jewish, nor because he lacks competence, but simply because he has shown sympathy for Quebec, for sovereignists and for French-speaking people: "Like a dog, he is accused of being rabid." That Levine should be pilloried on the basis of his belonging to a group—is that not racist? asks Nuovo.

> Isn't this discrimination contrary to the ideas of humanity, justice, fraternity, dignity and equality that Canada has always boasted about? … The Levine affair, backed by the stupidity of Stéphane Dion, by the crass demagogy of Mike Harris who openly aligns himself with his population, and above all by the hypocritical silence of Chrétien and Copps who, however, never miss an opportunity to give us a tirade on bilingualism and grand liberal principles, is an attack on moral conscience.

Nuovo concludes by commenting that to his knowledge, Levine had not been booed while head of a French-Catholic hospital in Montreal, nor were proceedings instituted against him in the court of public opinion.

Le Droit. *Le Droit* gives front-page, banner headline treatment to Mike Harris's statement: "Harris opposed to Levine," with the subhead, "The Premier of Ontario, Mike Harris, squarely condemned the decision to give the post of chief executive officer of the Ottawa Hospital to David Levine." In the lead paragraph, Jules Richer of Canadian Press reports that in Mike Harris's assessment, Quebec sovereignists have no place in the public administration of Ontario. "I believe that we prefer that people paid with tax dollars should be interested in keeping the country united," Harris said in Toronto.

Inside the paper, a prominent story notes the support of Liberal MPP Dalton McGuinty for Levine. McGuinty is quoted as saying that one should distinguish political opinions from the ability to do a job: "Mr. Levine was hired to run a hospital, not a country." Are we about to start asking potential public servants, in a way reminiscent of McCarthy in the United States, "Are you, or have you ever been, a separatist?"

Another story draws attention to hospital employees who wish the affair would soon be over so that the task of caring for patients and the details of amalgamation can be addressed. Barry Butler and Ted Zuara, pictured in a photograph, are quoted as saying that David Levine would not be able to work amid this hostile opposition, while a cartoon depicts a man looking at an "H" sign and wondering whether it stood for "Hostility, Hatred, Hysteria" or "Hargne" (a French word for "spite").

An editorial by *Le Droit* publisher, Pierre Bergeron, wonders what would have happened at Tuesday night's meeting if David Levine had been brought in, led by the nose, like a "bad scene in a western movie": "Let's fervently wish that the shameful display of intolerance, intransigence and racism before the Hospital board Tuesday evening, was nothing more than an unhealthy release for frustrated people suffering from strong feelings." If the frothing of a minority reflected the feelings of the majority "we would have reason to worry and the government would have reason to raise serious questions about the mental health of our society and of its democratic institutions."

The editorial wisely recounts important details of recent history that have produced strong emotions. The demonstration of intolerance and incomprehension, Bergeron writes, is the final explosion at the end of a silent period, during which the majority were never able to digest the reorganization of health care in the region, the spectacular survival campaign for the Montfort Hospital, the insistence on the necessity for services in French and the closing of the two big health institutions in the capital. "If you mix into all of this the orneriness of those who could never swallow their cereal with French written on the package, you get to see the totally useless psychodramas which cause our society to regress, deflecting it from its ends and diminishing all of us in our humanity." The most troubling aspect of the sad affair, concludes Bergeron, is that in mixing up business and politics, little by little we lose the illusions of openness and tolerance with which we have been cradled "in the shadow of the Canadian Parliament."

A letter by Jean-Paul Perreault, president of Impératif français, argues that fundamental human rights are being threatened in Canada by the "extreme and racist reaction" against Levine because of his political past. The letter quotes from the United Nations Universal Declaration of Rights, articles 2, 7, 19 and 21, suggesting that Stéphane Dion re-read some of his father's writings and political science textbooks explaining the Declaration. The letter appears to have been written without knowledge of some of the quotations from Stéphane Dion carried in Pierre O'Neill's May 21 article in *Le Devoir*.

Ottawa Citizen. The *Ottawa Citizen* puts Suharto's resignation upfront but places a Levine story in a prominent top right-hand column with the headline "Harris: Levine wrong choice." Richard Brennan and Tim Naumetz write: "Toronto—The Ottawa Hospital would have been better off hiring a foreigner to head up its newly amalgamated operation than a known separatist, Premier Mike Harris said yesterday." Harris is quoted as saying on radio: "Given that background, and if that's what he still believes in, he wouldn't have been our first choice. Surely there is administrative capability within Ontario, or [at] least a Canadian or even a non-Canadian who believes in Canada and in keeping Canada together."

The story later reports that former premiers, Bill Davis, David Peterson and Bob Rae, "urged Mr. Harris to tone down the rhetoric over Mr. Levine's appointment." Peterson is quoted: "I don't discriminate against a man on the basis of his politics, any more than I would on the basis of his colour or religion." Likewise Rae says: "You never divide the province on language or religion. It's essential that you not take sides, but stay in a position where you can be a voice of moderation." A further quotation from Premier Harris puts the phrase "with the people" in a context which gives a different impression from that conveyed in *Le Droit's* cartoon mentioned earlier.

"How they [the board] spend their money [$330,000 a year on Levine's salary] ... is really none of the business of the province of Ontario, but I'm with the people, I would like an explanation as to how this makes sense." To say you are "with the people" means one thing when related to the angry mob shouting anti-French insults, and another thing when linked only to the demand for an explanation of the board's actions. Mr. Harris is also quoted as saying: "I would rather have somebody who is not a separatist ... I can't do anything about it ... on the other hand, residents of Ontario have said they are concerned that taxpayer dollars are funding relatively well-paid positions ... for somebody they believe is not interested in keeping the country together." The quotation encourages an anti-separatist mentality, but not as categorically as some French accounts made it appear.

The story quotes Liberal leader Dalton McGuinty's remark that it would be wrong to discriminate against a person based on their political views. Prime Minister Jean Chrétien is quoted as telling a news conference in Rome, where he was on a trade mission, that "In Canada, political considerations are not a question that we ask for employment."[5] Deborah Grey, deputy parliamentary leader of the Reform party, is described as an unexpected ally of Levine: "Nobody should ever be fired for their political beliefs," the story quotes her as saying.

Inside, *Citizen* columnist Janice Kennedy writes of her strong revulsion against the "howling mob of self-proclaimed patriots" who "took over a public meeting intended to answer questions about the controversial hiring of David Levine." "Is it too late to apply for foreign citizenship? I'll take anything, as long as it's not Canadian. Not this week. Not after Tuesday night's spectacle in Ottawa. Not after Sunday's in Montreal." This final phrase refers to convicted FLQ terrorist Raymond Villeneuve and his association, which distributed two-page letters door-to-door in Westmount to reminded the reader that "today is the 35th anniversary of the mailbox operation in Westmount, conducted by the Front de Libération du Québec, on May 17, 1963: 10 bombs, five explosions, one Canadian army officer seriously wounded." The letter warned what life might be like if Westmount opted for partition from a separate Quebec.

The *Citizen* carries both an editorial and a column by the publisher, Russell Mills. The editorial, "To move forward," maintains that David Levine "should not become the chief executive officer of Ottawa's new megahospital" but dissociates the *Citizen* from the harassment and intimidation of Tuesday's meeting. Mills blames the appointed and inexperienced board for the whole problem, saying that members might "stand by their original decision, in which case they must ask themselves whether they can in good conscience continue on as public trustees, which in effect is what they are." The editorial put a large part of the responsibility for "the board's costly mistake" on Nick Mulder, the hospital board chair. "It seems unlikely that the board can regain public confidence under his chairmanship." Mills sees Levine's job as being "as much political as administrative": "Levine may be a superb administrator [but] his history as a separatist candidate disqualifies him for the equally important political component of the job in Ottawa."

A story in the front page of the *Citizen's* City section analyses, with the help of pollster Conrad Winn, the type of person who spoke out against Levine at Tuesday's meeting. According to Winn the people may have been old and angry, but that's because they are informed, are truly concerned about the future of health care, and are riding the populist wave of Canadian discontent.

The *Citizen's* full page of letters appears under the non-committal heading: "The Levine affair: Readers speak out." Eight out of twelve of these letters are pro-Levine. Don Francis of Chelsea submits a strongly-worded attack on MPP Garry Guzzo, describing his campaign as a "very serious threat to the liberties of all Canadians … [that] adds fuel to nationalistic flames all around us." Federalists might experience comparable treatment in Quebec. "It does not take a lot of little battles like those to weaken the sense of national purpose that still thrives throughout Canada." He describes the resentment displayed by Mr. Guzzo's followers as the "mirror image" of the same desperate measures proposed by separatists. Alastair Mullin of Ottawa envisages Garry Guzzo and others setting up a Committee on UnCanadian Activities. Maybe, while the politicians are busy, "we can let the hospital hire the best qualified candidate for the job, and start to repair the hatchet job successive governments have done on our health-care system."

Len Gelfand of Ottawa denies that separatists are interested in breaking up Canada, any more than an adolescent who leaves home is interested in breaking up the family. "Separatists are minor contributors to the breakup of Canada compared to those who denigrate government and demand its reduction." Jane Hilliard of Renfrew wonders what happened to freedom of speech, thought and association. She does not believe Levine would use the Ottawa Hospital as a forum for a separatist agenda.

Bob Fitzgerald of Ottawa complains that the *Citizen* has repeatedly crossed the line that distinguishes *reporting* the news from *manufacturing* it: "The inflammatory and ill-considered headlines are certainly the most egregious aspect of this campaign to stir up public opinion. Is it really front-page news that 'a separatist' or 'the PQ's envoy' has been appointed to administer a hospital?" He suggests that the *Citizen* could hardly believe that Levine would "deliber-

ately mismanage the affairs of the hospital in order to harm Ontario and federalism? ... How can his political affiliations (past or present) be relevant to his
selection for this position?" Fitzgerald also blames the *Citizen* for giving so
much attention to MPP Garry Guzzo's "foolish and intemperate remarks": "The
front-page headline 'Levine won't resign' (implying that he should) is but one
more example of this approach." The *Citizen* has shown some "appallingly
poor judgement" by its headlines and much of its reporting. It was "embarrassing and deeply disappointing" that Ottawa's main English-language newspaper has "chosen to lead this misguided movement [against Levine] rather than
simply reporting on it or, better yet, denouncing it."[6]

Siobhan Stein of Ottawa holds that David Levine's qualifications are impeccable and that the intolerance shown him leads to destruction, fear and racism: "We waved our flags in a referendum in the name of tolerance and acceptance," but the reaction to Levine revealed hypocrisy. It showed "that we were
not sincere in our approach to Quebec, that it was all for the show." She apolo-
gizes to Levine.

Of the letters opposed to Levine, Ottawan George Coleman admonishes
Levine for not saying clearly, when he had the chance, that he was a federalist.
Brian Cayen, also of Ottawa, declares that "separatists are enemies of this country and should be treated with the disdain and disgust that goes with that position." He advocates terminating Levine's appointment and demanding the resignation of the board. Patricia and Calvin Kempffer could not trust in anyone
who has such poor judgement as to belong to and work for the separatist government of Quebec. Finally, Juris Mazutis of Nepean asks why half a million
non-francophones left Quebec if the Quebec Charter of Rights gave the protec-
tions described by Gilles Duceppe. Pro-Canada sentiments were enough,
Mazutis claims, to "disqualify any candidate from employment in the Quebec
public service," and English hospitals were being shut down in Quebec. In that
light, it did not seem right to lean over backwards to be "fair" in Ontario. If we
pay the bill we should not have to support those whose views are diametrically
opposite to ours on an issue as basic as national unity, he writes.

Ottawa Sun. The *Ottawa Sun* has a front-page headline, double inside-page
coverage, two columns and four letters all devoted to the Levine affair. The
headline "Levine battle rages" in inch-high type is sandwiched between two
smaller headings: "Board debates fate of 'separatist' CEO" and "PM says hospital boss shouldn't be fired," a story about Prime Minister Chrétien wading into
the "rough waters of the Ottawa Hospital debate, saying embattled CEO David
Levine should not be turfed because of his PQ ties." The next paragraph cites
an opposing quotation from the CEO of Toronto's Sick Kids Hospital, Mike
Strofolino: "Decisions are influenced by politics. Politics will always play a
role."

Earl McRae urges people to keep up the protest in a column headed "Don't let patriot fires go out under Levine." "Keep the heat on," he advises. "Let them know that if it's civil disobedience they want, civil disobedience they'll get, because there are times and circumstances in the affairs of a nation when civil disobedience is proper and honorable for a great cause." He specifically suggests a boycott of Bell Canada if board chair Nick Mulder does not resign. He identifies Mulder as president and CEO of Stentor Telecom Policy, a lobbying arm of Bell.

McRae argues that Levine's separatism should have been an issue, that the nine-member search committee should have presented the board with some choices and that the board should have followed better its terms of reference, including having "an awareness of and the ability to build and facilitate *strong public and community relationships*" (original emphasis). He questions whether the current board, "given the Levine Lunacy," fit the Ottawa Hospital Administrative Bylaw definition as one that is "seen by the population served as *capable, experienced, and well able to lead the Hospital.*" He accuses Ontario Health Minister Elizabeth Witmer of "political cowardice" for not using the power of the Ontario Public Hospitals Act to reverse the Levine hiring, and urges his readers to "Keep on fighting."

The first page of the *Sun's* two-page inside spread is headed "Workers fear losing jobs," with the subhead "Anglophone hospital employees worry about Levine's administration." Stephanie Rubec begins her story: "Fear is rippling through the Ottawa Hospital as employees worry about what type of leader David Levine will be if he takes over as CEO." Ontario Nurses Association spokeswoman Barb LeBlanc says that anglophone nurses are now even more "worried they'll lose their jobs during the amalgamation if their French is not up to par," a longtime fear that was heightened by the thought that Levine might maintain strong ties with Quebec and favour French nurses. A second story mentions Prime Minister Chrétien's defence of Levine, which has already been described.

On the facing page, a picture of be-medalled Daniel O'Dwyer, shown receiving a standing ovation at the Tuesday evening meeting, is headlined "Hospital board looks at hiring." The subhead quotes Judy Brown, public affairs officer for the Civic site of the Ottawa Hospital, saying, "It's a very important discussion."

Donna Casey reports some of the board members' reactions to Tuesday's meeting, including that of trustee Pierre de Blois: "Had it been in the 1890s people would have been lynched." He felt that the explosive meeting convinced more board members to stick to their decision rather than give in to that mob mentality. Trustee Maria Barrados is quoted as saying, "I think it would be irresponsible for us all to resign."

Ron Corbett writes in his column that he detests the separatists but is unwilling to condone depriving even one Canadian of the right to free speech. He denounces the way the crowd shouted down Ottawa-Vanier MP Mauril Bélanger at the Tuesday meeting: "The crowd gathered at the Civic Hospital drowned out such people with heckles and catcalls. They applauded their achievement." He was not going to defend the Levine appointment, but the right to free speech is something "we fight wars for." "I'm not giving it up for a hospital administrator," he concludes.

Three of four letters published are opposed to Levine. Reuel S. Amdur corrects a misquotation by Earl McRae. He had not defined patriotism, as had Samuel Johnson, as the "last resort of a scoundrel." Amdur says that he defined patriotism as "the first resort of a scoundrel, as had Ambrose Bierce." Nurse Fran Monaghan expresses her fear that Levine will promote the French language in the area hospitals: "And therefore some of these employees are going to come from Quebec and provide us with more separatist ideas."

Friday, May 22

This day was particularly significant for the print media, as it was the first opportunity to report on the previous day's press conference in which the Ottawa Hospital board announced its intention to reaffirm its hiring of David Levine, a household name in the Ottawa area.

Ottawa Citizen. The *Ottawa Citizen* devotes nearly four full news pages and most of the front section editorial page to this hot item that has captured public attention. The City section carries an additional full page of letters and two columns on the editorial page.

The front-page story, by Daniel Leblanc, has a banner headline: "Levine was once a Liberal, too," which forcefully contradicts the not uncommon notion that Levine was a diehard separatist out to promote his political views. If he could be shown to have changed political affiliations, this would make him into a careerist rather than a separatist with a political agenda. The story is based on a statement by Serge Ménard, a "prominent Montreal Liberal who sold a party membership to Mr. Levine in the late 1980s," that Levine once confided to him that he believed Quebec would never separate from Canada. Ménard, "a member of the board of directors of Verdun Hospital in Montreal when Mr. Levine ran the institution in the 1980s," was asked by then-Premier Robert Bourassa to "keep an eye on Mr. Levine because of fears that he would load the hospital administration with separatists. Mr. Ménard says that never happened. In fact, once, over a meal, Mr. Levine appeared to renounce his PQ past."

This story has a powerful impact. So much of the haranguing of Mr. Levine was based on the preconception that he was a "rabid" (to use Lowell Green's term) separatist. This new information called that notion seriously into question. According to Ménard, Levine joined the PQ because of its social-democratic agenda, and not to achieve separation.

The second story, written by Mark Gollom and headed "Defiant board stands by its man," recounts the Ottawa Hospital Board's decision on the previous day to stand behind Levine who is to begin his new job ahead of time, on June 15. Chair Nick Mulder said that the board would not discriminate on the basis of his political affiliation. Another board member, Sol Sinder, drew attention to the problem of obtaining another suitable candidate if Levine were fired, and the harm to health care in the region from the delay. Mulder admitted that the anger of the community had not been anticipated: "We apologize to the community for inadvertently opening wounds on the serious issue of Canadian unity." The board had "received hundreds of calls of support, including promises of financial contributions from people who have never donated before," Mulder was quoted as saying. A 7 inch by 7 inch photograph of him accompanied the story.

The third story, by Randy Boswell, focused on one of the groups protesting the Levine appointment, Solidarité Outaouais Solidarity. The leader of this group, Dany Gravel, said the firestorm of controversy "will one day be viewed as a 'watershed' in the national unity debate": "We have been expected to tolerate everything. But the people, on Tuesday, decided to send a message that there will be no more free lunch at the Canadian table. Unfortunately, the board did not hear them." Boswell notes that CFRA radio talk-show host Lowell Green said that he was "in a state of absolute shock" at the board's decision to retain Levine.

A page-two story by Christopher Guly gives a roundup of reaction in the press across Canada. Guly writes that the reaction in *Le Soleil* to the Tuesday meeting was one of shock, according to editorial page writer Donald Charette: "A lot of people were shocked by the hostile reaction, attitude and tone. Even federalists were quite shocked." The *Montreal Gazette* saw the affair as a display of McCarthyism. But the radio station CJAD had many people calling for Levine's head. In selected Vancouver, Winnipeg and Edmonton papers, the story had not yet attracted much attention, Guly reported.

At the top of page three a general rubric, "The Levine Controversy" precedes four stories. The first and largest, by Daniel Leblanc, is headed "A maverick from the start," with the large-type summary: "The Ottawa Hospital's new administrator is a rarity in many ways: an anglophone who supported Quebec sovereignty, and a remarkable health care executive." A 6 inch by 9 inch picture of a thoughtful looking, bearded Levine accompanies the text. The story is very favourable to Levine, countering typical misconceptions: "David Levine is an exception to the rule," he writes. "His destiny, as an anglophone from Montreal's Jewish community, was to become an unconditional lover of Canada." Exposure at university to separatist ideas in the late '60s and early '70s changed his views. He became one of a few dozen idealists ready to give the PQ a chance in the light of their progressive social policies. Leblanc notes that another anglophone who followed the same path was David Payne, now a Quebec MNA, who said, "We never perceived the PQ to have a platform to oppress the English. We saw Bill 101 as an attempt to redress imbalances of the past or to protect, promote and encourage the use of the French language. Serge Ménard is quoted as saying that he was told to watch Levine in case he tried to load the hospital with other *péquistes:* "It never happened. Yes, he loaded the hospital, but only with the best possible people." The chair of the Notre-Dame Hospital in Montreal, André Bisson, also spoke in superlative terms about Levine, according to Leblanc, describing him as a tireless worker who thinks, lives and breathes health care and as "the best hospital administrator in Canada." Leblanc's account makes Levine out to be a gifted human being rather than a doctrinaire, agenda-following politician. Had it been published a few weeks earlier, it would have done much to lower the temperature of the controversy.

Two other stories on page three stem from an interview by writer Jeremy Mercer with the executive research firm that recommended David Levine, Korn Ferry: "Headhunters who found Levine say board made right choice" and "Dismissal may be possible without financial penalty"; the latter story explores the board's possible outs with a labour lawyer.

Luiza Chwialkowska's page four profile of Nick Mulder characterizes him as a resolute, courageous person accustomed to making tough decisions and sticking with them. Former Supply and Services Minister Paul Dick spoke of his "solid judgement" and added, "He's very bright, very capable." Mulder was Dick's deputy minister of supply and services from 1990 to 1993. Another story explores backgrounds of unsuccessful candidates for the Ottawa Hospital position. A fourth piece reports Ottawa-Carleton regional chair Bob Chiarelli as saying that the David Levine "debacle" is proof that the provincial health care system needs to be overhauled. Without coming down for or against the Levine appointment, Chiarelli attacked the process: "We were left with a spectacle of an ad hoc meeting called to deal with a health care issue that was very emotional and divisive in the community." He called for good communication and cooperation between Queens Park and the health-care field in Ottawa-Carleton and other regions.

On the editorial page, a column by John Robson, headed "Why David Levine has got to go" argues that Levine is unsuitable because he holds views that are deeply offensive to the community. "Like separatism," he writes.

Susan Riley argues in her column that the Levine decision was "badly bungled—particularly by not introducing Levine at once—but it would have been completely unprincipled had it abandoned him now." She has changed her view since the previous column and explains: "What I was doing—what some opponents of the appointment may still be doing—is misdirecting accumulated anger with Lucien Bouchard, Jacques Parizeau, Gilles Duceppe and a legion of less sovereigntist leaders towards Levine." She now sees that eliminating Levine from contention on the basis of his political beliefs "would be a betrayal of the Canadian values, including tolerance, that we say we cherish."

She differentiated the case of Jean-Louis Roux, who had a youthful flirtation with the Nazis, from Levine's case, which involved commitment to a legitimate political party and not a violent, racist organization.

The full page of letters is headed, again noncommittally, "Responses to 'mob' at Levine hearing," and the letters run about 7–5 in favour of Levine. Irving Altman of Nepean, Catherine Johnston of Ottawa and Lorne Trottier of Dorval argue that Levine's political beliefs are irrelevant and that he should be given a chance to prove himself. Trottier says that her company "would be much poorer if we hired and promoted only people with politically correct views." Jean-Marie Joly of Ottawa wonders why the *Citizen* does not investigate Levine's past performance in Montreal. Simon Segal of Ottawa comments that the media has done "their usual hatchet job" and has influenced a number of people's thinking about the David Levine appointment. Many of those who came to Tuesday's meeting "came prepared not to listen, as was evidenced by the catcalls and interruptions for those who spoke for Levine," he writes.

Letters opposed to Levine make the familiar claims about the undeservingness or the threat of a separatist holding a government job in Ottawa. One of the letters opposed is signed Dr. Marguerite E. Ritchie, President, Human Rights Institute of Canada, who gives a pejorative connotation to a statement by Levine. Levine is quoted as saying, "This is a wonderful opportunity to show that the two founding nations of Canada can work together, and come up with one of the great institutions of Canada." This, to Ritchie, implies another experiment in the 50–50 sawing up of Canada outside Quebec: "I don't want to have to go to a hospital that is being experimented on to show that two founding nations can work together." She congratulates Ottawans for opposing Levine and adds, "Nobody should be in charge of the reorganization of the hospitals if he believes in the false separatist teaching of two nations."

Kent Glowinski thinks people "should be openly embracing [Levine's] appointment as a way to show how open and flexible the Canadian federation is to all ranges of political views, even ones that try to destroy the nation."

Bob Fitzgerald criticizes the *Citizen* for its poll about Levine, saying that it omitted the important question: "Do you agree (disagree) that Canadians may be denied employment on the basis of their political beliefs." Fitzgerald notes that, in phrasing certain questions, the poll implanted ideas that people probably did not already have; for example, people were asked to agree or disagree with the statement "a separatist cannot be fair and objective dealing with Quebec, whose government pays less than the full cost of the services that Ottawa hospitals give to Quebec residents." All in all, however, the *Citizen* cast Levine in a much more favourable light than hitherto.

Ottawa Sun. The *Ottawa Sun* sports the front-page banner headline "Levine stays put" with the subhead "Ottawa Hospital board stands by former separatist candidate." The story states that the board has decided to stick with the decision to hire David Levine as CEO, though it apologizes to the public for not being prepared for the fallout and not doing a better job of selling Levine.

Inside, on page four, a story by Stephanie Rubec proclaims that the fight to oust Levine has been lost. The banner headline is a quotation from Regional Chair Bob Chiarelli, "It's time for healing," and the lead sentence reads simply "David Levine is here to stay." At the centre-top is a 4 inch by 6 inch photograph of a composed, pensive Nick Mulder, accompanied by excerpts from the board's statement:

> Mr. Levine's hiring has caused a reaction among some members of our community that, clearly, we did not fully anticipate. We apologize to the community for inadvertently opening wounds on the serious issue of Canadian unity. We commit to you that we will work diligently to earn your trust and respect. Our mission and primary interest are to make the Ottawa Hospital the best hospital in Canada.

A further story recounts how David Levine backed out from introducing Quebec Premier Lucien Bouchard's address to a Philadelphia business luncheon on May 21. Levine, still delegate general to New York, decided to stay in New York. Keith Henderson, president of Montreal's Equality Party, told the *Sun:* "Obviously, he backed out because of all the fuss .... The man should never have been hired. Obviously he is very political if he was called on to introduce Bouchard."

In his column Earl McRae interprets the swift decision of the board to retain Levine as an in-your-face reaction to the "howling mob"—a description given to the Tuesday night crowd by "pro-Levine weeping hearts, including some in the media." What he didn't say is that even people who were opposed to the Levine appointment were embarrassed by the intolerant reaction. McRae defines "Howling mob" as "their coda *(sic)*" for "Bigots, Racists, Rednecks, Ignoramuses." Having been perhaps instigator-in-chief, McRae was not going to let them hang out to dry: "First of all, you were far from a 'howling mob.' You are Canadians who believe in Canada, and if your deep pro-Canada, anti-destroyers emotionalism leads to shouting down the separatist appeasers, good for your Maple Leaf hearts."

Ron Corbett reflects the mood of the news stories. "Battle over, let's get on with life" was the heading for his column. He thought that a "victory" had been won by the Levine protestors: "If there was ever any doubt about how passionately people in Ottawa feel about this country, about how visceral Canada is to us in the nation's capital, about what we're willing to do to defend it—I think those doubts have been erased."

Apprehensions were kept alive with a page-five news story headed "Bilingualism draft puts staff on alert":

> A draft copy of an Ottawa Hospital policy on bilingualism dictating levels of French proficiency for every staff position has employees scared for their future .... The draft confirms their biggest fear: Employees from cashier to nurse need to speak some French to work at the amalgamated hospital.

But Jean Leroux, a trustee of the Ottawa Hospital, said that only a certain percentage of staff in each department would need to speak French and that, with nurses turning to the U.S. for jobs, they would not want a policy that would force more health care workers out.

The *Sun's* editorial "Consequences" was a scathing condemnation of the board's decision to retain Levine. "Damn the consequences to the community that has become dangerously and perhaps irreparably divided by a controversy that should never have been allowed to happen." The issue would not go away, the *Sun* writes. "It will linger like a festering wound for months, possibly years, undermining public support for an important community institution."

Steve Madely also devotes part of his column to Levine, humorously sending up the worst fears of the anti-Levine extremists. Watch out, now, for the following, he says:

> The doctors visiting your ward ask ... How do you feel about the right of Quebec to pursue its destiny? ... All the apostrophes disappear from hospital signs .... They won't take a blood sample unless you can prove it has been "pure laine" for six generations .... No maple leaf desk flags are allowed on your bedside table .... Heart surgeon Dr. Wilburt Keon has been ordered to get rid of his car and buy a Peugot *(sic)*.

A full page of letters was devoted to Levine, accompanied by a reprint of the cartoon showing Levine entering his new office, saying, "Actually ... I'd *prefer* my office to be in a *separate* building." The letters are 6-4 in favour of Levine, with one noncommittal. The lead letter and the letter of the day are both anti-Levine. Art Turner of Ottawa makes the point that the Liberal government appoints Liberal senators, Liberal judges and party hacks to patronage jobs. Therefore it is nonsense for Liberal MP Mauril Bélanger to say that one cannot discriminate on the basis of political beliefs when offering employment. Turner says he is not going to give money to a hospital that hires Levine.

Jean-Pierre Picard, of Hull, contrasts the "We love you" march in Montreal on the eve of the October 1995 referendum with the bigotry of those who "judge that half of the Quebec population is not suited for a job in Canada." "It is through the same stupidity and shortsightedness that Louis Riel ended up being hanged," he concludes.

Kent Glowinski says that "we should be openly embracing [Levine's] appointment as a way to show how open and flexible the Canadian federation is to all ranges of political views, even ones which try to destroy the nation." (The same letter, with slightly different editing, appears in the *Citizen* on May 22 and the *Sun* on May 23. In the *Citizen* but not the *Sun*, Glowinski identifies himself as Montreal 1997 Progressive Conservative candidate, Skeena riding.) Raynald Adams says he does not believe that "a violation of David Levine's rights is 'the price he should pay for his political beliefs.' If David Levine loses his job, Quebecers will need no further proof that English Canada values human rights no more than your average dictatorship, and I, for one, anxiously await its future sermons on Quebec's 'intolerance.'"

Dominque Auger detects a contradiction between the *Sun's* position regarding the hiring policies under the Rae government, namely that competence alone should decide, and its policy regarding the hiring of Levine. The *Sun* appends a note saying that Auger is mixing apples and oranges, because the Rae government's work on affirmative action is different from the Levine case.

Philip Bury writes that firing Levine would be a "gross injustice, ... shame our community, Ontario and Canada" and help Bouchard and Parizeau prove that Ontario hates Quebec. "Firing David Levine would help separatism and help break up Canada. Those who claim they oppose him for patriotic reasons should think about this. Leave him alone. Let him do his job." To this the *Sun* appends the lame note: "It's not that simple."

J. Narraway says that he did not "recall the supporters for Levine rallying to the cause of the trampled rights of non-separatists in the supposed democratic province of Quebec." One should point out in answer to Narraway that there are some highly visible defenders of the rights of non-separatists in Quebec. William Johnson, the new head of Alliance Quebec, did support Levine's right to retain his position when I interviewed him on the question early in June 1998.

Le Journal de Montréal. The Montreal French language press has become intensely interested in the Levine affair. A full page *Journal de Montréal* story by Laurent Soumis is headed "David Levine keeps his job," characterizing him as the best person for the job, one who would not be able to use his position to look after his political interests. Soumis notes that Quebec Liberal leader Jean Charest was informed about the decision in time for the 6 p.m. television news, where he said that the decision revealed that "Canada works, as our history shows."

In a separate story, headed "After the hysteria against David Levine, the wave extends to francophones," Soumis writes: "While the competence of francophone doctors and the relevance of health care in French is publicly put in question, the anglophone dailies are calling for civil disobedience and squarely advocating intolerance." Reference to "the anglophone dailies" gives the impression that the call for civil disobedience is widely shared, but columnist Earl McRae, who advocated such action, can hardly be said to represent the viewpoint of the *Sun*, let alone the "anglophone dailies."

Soumis also reports that the anglophone dailies had published numerous letters in favour of giving Levine the "punishment for traitors" and calling for the definite abandonment of a "language which is in decline." Some denounced the hiring of "less qualified" medical staff who were bilingual.

Jean Chrétien and Stéphane Dion are recognized as having "tardily" appealed to reason, not in time to prevent Ottawa Mayor Jim Watson from calling for Levine's dismissal nor for preventing Ottawa-Carleton regional chair Bob Chiarelli from suggesting that Levine renounce his separatist views in writing, Soumis writes. The head of the Fédération des communautés francophones et acadienne, Gino LeBlanc, is quoted as saying that the disgraceful treatment of David Levine forebodes nothing good for the unity of the country, coming after three difficult years for Ontario francophones.

Le Droit. Le Droit by contrast stresses the positive side of the board's decision with the front-page banner headline "Levine in position June 15" and the overline "The Ottawa Hospital board refuses to yield to pressure from his detractors." Most of the front page shows an earnest looking Nick Mulder, hands forward and upturned, confirming Levine's appointment at a press conference. The summary of the story by Isabelle Ducas reads: "The Hospital board did not yield to pressure from citizens who, for three weeks, have called with anger and venom for the resignation of David Levine from his post of CEO of the institution: it announced yesterday that it would maintain its decision to hire 'the person most qualified to occupy the position.'"

The story quotes board member Jean Leroux as saying that the reasons for choosing Levine might have been conveyed to the public from the beginning, but that various forces at work were revealed during the controversy:

> It seemed as though at bottom it was a debate on national unity but it should be realised that the restructuring process imposed by the Harris government has not brought unanimity either in the board or the community. There are forces seeking to destabilize us, and Mr. Levine has become a lightning rod for those forces. But I'm proud we resisted them.

He and other francophone board members said they were "shaken," in Leroux's words, by what transpired Tuesday: "I've worked for a long time in the community and I've never seen anything so low. It was disgraceful and disgusting, but it was not representative of the community I know."

Inside *Le Droit* a headline proclaimed "Observers heave a sigh of relief," and Annie Morin reported that the majority of political observers questioned by the newspaper were relieved to learn of the Ottawa Hospital board's decision to keep Levine. Vanier mayor Guy Cousineau was reported as saying that francophones were big winners in the decision. Ottawa Mayor Jim Watson and MPP Garry Guzzo were said not to have "deigned" to return repeated phone calls from the newspaper.

Another story, by Paul Gaboury, reports that the Montfort Hospital administration is not afraid of a backlash from the decision. Michel Gratton, spokesperson for the hospital, notes that since Tuesday the anti-Levine voices repeat that they are not anti-francophone and that they all want to save the country, so we should not worry about the Montfort.

A clever cartoon that takes a dig at Mike Harris depicts him on all fours next to howling wolves, saying "I'm with the people." As earlier remarked, the words are taken out of context to give a different impression.

Le Droit's editorial, by Murray Maltais is headed "An upright board"; the subhead reads "Intimidation should never become a form of government." Maltais congratulates the board for not "yielding to blackmail and intimidation":

> Shame, yes shame on the Ontario Premier. He has always refused comment on the decision to close the Montfort Hospital. But on Wednesday he did not hesitate a second to range himself on the side of those who did not want David Levine as CEO of the new Ottawa Hospital, because of the latter's sovereignist sympathies.

Maltais draws attention to the fact that Ottawa is part of a national capital region.

> The Levine affair is not a separatist matter. It is a linguistic one. In Canada's capital the francophone population forms a third of the clientele for the new Ottawa Hospital. Who wants to see a scandalous denial of the right to be treated in French, or to die in one's own language? The situation, blown out of all proportion by demogoguery and the media for their purposes, has been brought back to its proper dimensions. It shows just how far fear and ignorance can be manipulated to distort the debate and intimidate the undecided.

He notes that the board was divided, despite the show of unanimity in its decision, and that the procedure for choosing Levine remains a source of uneasiness; the board should have been presented with alternatives by the selection committee, he says. The editorial concludes that Franco-Ontarians should be on the watch for trouble, with the Ontario premier having demonstrated his willingness to shape his opinions after those who claim to represent the majority.

Another inside story reports with a banner headline: "The National Assembly condemns the intolerance towards Levine." The Quebec legislature voted unanimously to denounce the intolerance toward Levine, and reiterated "the importance of respecting, in our democratic society, the fundamental principle of freedom of opinion." The story, by Michel Hébert of the Canadian Press, also quotes Quebec Premier Lucien Bouchard from Philadelphia: "In all he's done, Mr. Levine has only left behind compliments, praise and great achievements. He is a great Quebecer." Bouchard said he found it "totally sad" to see what had happened and retained from the episode that "there was some distance to travel on the side of tolerance."

On its letters page *Le Droit* publishes the full text of what Ottawa-Vanier MP Mauril Bélanger tried to communicate at Tuesday's meeting before he was shouted down. He reminds readers that he was one of the organizers of the big federalist pre-referendum rally in Montreal, and that he also launched a defence, with the support of the *Sun*, for those who were prosecuted in Quebec for violating the Elections Act during the rally and who thus had their legal costs defrayed. He notes that there is general unanimity that whoever occupies the Ottawa Hospital job should check their political opinions at the office door:

> David Levine has repeated on many occasions that he would do so. We all have rights in this country and they apply to everybody, including separatists. We cannot discriminate against or dismiss anyone by reason of their political convictions. Acting this way would lead us to unstable and dangerous ground. It would go against the fundamental values shared by Canadians: democracy, fundamental freedoms and tolerance.
>
> Separatists are people like anyone else and should be treated as such. They are our neighbours, citizens like us, sometimes our kin, our colleagues, our brothers and sisters. They have opinions which seem to us out of place or without foundation, but it remains nevertheless that they have a right to these opinions. We will never change them by resorting to coercion. If we want the separatists to fall in line with our view, and we should assure ourselves whether we want to resolve this incessant problem, we will settle nothing by treating them in the way some have wanted to treat David Levine. We will never convince them with that attitude. We can hardly expect another to adopt our point of view if we don't show openness of mind and heart on our side, or if we exclude them. That would be far from a conciliatory approach.

To those willing to think about the question, Bélanger concludes, "I would like to leave you with these words: the way we treat those who have opinions different from or contrary to our own is the real challenge of a democracy. I hope that as a community we will be able to meet this challenge."

A second letter compares the Levine case to that of the Dreyfus affair 100 years ago. Daniel Chartrand of Vanier notes that in February 1898, Émile Zola found himself accused in court, his comments buried by inarticulate howls in a packed hall, the smell of a stifled massacre in the air, palpable hatred in people's eyes. "In short," said Chartrand, "everything we saw in the televised report of the Ottawa Hospital meeting last Tuesday."

Chartrand saw both cases as a witch-hunt, a parallel to McCarthyism:

> [The media] could play the holy untouchables while all the time stirring up the conflict. You only have to read the *Ottawa Sun* to note that in going for the lowest common denominator, you sell not a few papers.
>
> What disturbs me, what I find most distressing, is the type of anti-francophone baggage which has accompanied this affair. I think of the fellow who got up in an earlier press conference, complaining that there was too much French. This is the kind of person who, tears in his eyes, wants to know why sovereignists want sovereignty.
>
> When you can't take it out on francophones who aren't there, you have to beat up on whoever is on hand. The method is classical: in the name of a flashy patriotism, retrenched in one's infallibility, you are entitled to mow down whoever does not share your values, opinions, party, or language. As Samuel Johnson said (with proof Tuesday evening) "Patriotism is the last refuge of a scoundrel."
>
> These people, these "patriots" who cannot bear any talk other than their own, make me afraid. It's a patriotism that reeks, that denies the values of our country. It's a patriotism that distinguishes between "them" and "us."
>
> We should realize that those who take aim at Levine take aim at Franco-Ontarians. Zola was a "Dreyfusard." I am a "Levinard."
>
> I am Franco-Ontarian, a convinced federalist. It may sound quaint, but I love my country, I am a "patriot" in my own way. But I have to say that when I see something like Tuesday evening's display, I can't help thinking: yes, separatists, it's your game.

Le Devoir. *Le Devoir* gives the story prominence but with a very different emphasis from that of *Le Droit*. The front page headline reads "The Ottawa Hospital apologizes." The story stresses that although the board is sticking to its decision to hire Levine, it regrets having aroused fierce passions. The story also highlights the fact that the board feels it necessary to say that Levine will not be able to "make use of his position to champion his political interests."

Lise Bissonnette devotes a lengthy editorial to the Levine affair, under the heading "An idea of freedoms." In her view, the statements made by Ontario Premier Mike Harris in support of discrimination in hiring on the basis of political belief, much more than the hysterical gathering of furious citizens has transformed "the Levine affair" into a crisis of major importance. The hospital board decision to keep Levine, but shamefully to "apologize" to his opponents, was no doubt tied to this reprimand from on high and added to the uneasiness rather than dissipating it.

In Bissonnette's analysis of Tuesday's scene, the mob should not be considered a representative sample of the Ontario population. This type of meeting, she writes, attracts the most excited and excitable people: "In the old days, they rushed to public hangings; today they must content themselves with verbal lynchings, but their taste for muck is the same."

She faults the board for organizing the press conference, given the "open season" on separatists created by the popular press in Ottawa:

> How could one, if one really values Mr. Levine, expose him to such a display of public and degrading vindictiveness, which could jeopardise his own safety and even that of his family. Was the idea to appease the blackmailers, who will renew their demands now that they have received an apology? Idiocy is the mitigating circumstance for the shriekers, but those who open their way or yield to them are as much to blame, as Stéphane Dion understood too late, after having furnished by his "explanations" the pretext for crying traitor.

Bissonnette has especially harsh words for Premier Mike Harris:

> The turn taken by Harris was altogether of a different order, much more serious. Without being trapped, knowing perfectly the question in wait for him in a Toronto radio studio, the premier of Ontario declared Wednesday that he and the minister of health would have chosen not to hire Mr. Levine "*if he still believes in it,*" that is to say, in the sovereignty of Quebec. He came back to this in suggesting that a position paid for by public funds should be held only by people who believe in "Canadian unity" and that it would have been better to hire a "*non-Canadian who believes in Canada*" than a sovereignist like Mr. Levine, despite his being a Canadian.
>
> In short, not only did the premier of the most important Canadian province affirm that it is legitimate and proper to refuse to hire a person, based solely on his or her opinions, something that makes a mockery of the Canadian Charter of Rights and Freedoms, but it also suggests that sovereignists are not completely citizens, that they are in some way more foreign than foreigners, a new theory of internal xenophobia. The only reason why he did not overturn the decision to

hire Mr. Levine, he confided to his listeners, was that he did not have the power.

Bissonnette contrasts Harris's words with his supposed acceptance of the Calgary Declaration, the first line of which reads "All Canadians are equal and their rights are protected by law .... The diversity, tolerance, compassion and equality of opportunity offered by Canada are without equal in the world." The problem, as she sees it, is that the Canadian Charter of Rights has been used by different groups as a technical means to accomplish changes for their purposes. The letter of the law has been exploited,

> But its spirit, that of recognition of mutual freedoms, has had difficulty becoming embodied in the day-to-day. The Charter belongs to the juridical sphere more than the civic sphere, and that is how it happens that Mr. Harris, like the rioters who encourage him, probably doesn't grasp the enormity of the breach he proposes.
>
> The Levine affair is a time for assessing, for taking stock of this extraordinary gap between words and things, and rethinking the work of popular education, the deficiency of which is so evident today. What is gained by telling Canadians that their tolerance is "without equal in the world" when the reality, in the shadow of their federal Parliament, contradicts this assertion so coldly, an assertion which, incidentally, is insulting to all the democracies with which we are associated? It isn't an increase in Pharisaism that Canada needs in the face of the temptation to discriminate which arises. It needs a demanding discourse which gives citizens, instead of a haughty idea of themselves, a high idea of the freedoms which they must still learn to recognize and respect.

La Presse. *La Presse* gives a similar emphasis, proclaiming enthusiastically with a banner front-page headline "David Levine unanimously." The subhead states "The Ottawa Hospital maintains its decision; a Quebec motion condemns intolerance." Reporters Vincent Marissal and Chantal Hébert write:

> Resisting a strong movement against David Levine which is shaking the federal capital, the board of the new amalgamated Ottawa Hospital held fast to its position and entrusted the job of CEO to the former péquist candidate.
>
> Still shaken by the extremely virulent reaction of a few hundred people opposed to the nomination of a sovereignist to head their hospital, the board of directors cloaked its decision in apologies and promises to the population in the Ottawa region.

On an inside page *La Presse* devotes twelve column-inches of bold-faced type to the motion passed by the Quebec Legislature, which denounces intolerance towards Levine.

Toronto Star. The *Toronto Star* gives the story front-page coverage with a headline "Hospital backs CEO in unity uproar," and the subhead "Board stands behind ex-PQ candidate despite local outrage." The lead to the story by William Walker, the *Star's* Ottawa bureau chief, reads: "An Ottawa hospital board has apologized for opening national unity wounds but won't fire its newly appointed CEO over his past as a Parti Québécois candidate and supporter." In the fourth paragraph, Walker notes that "The Quebec media has widely reported the controversy as the worst anti-Quebec incident since the Brockville stomping of a Quebec flag." Apart from giving *Star* readers some of Levine's background, Walker interviews Second World War veteran Daniel O'Dwyer in his home, eliciting from him the remark that "You don't change a zebra's stripes. He won't change .... There's going to be more fire and more hate and more trouble. I'm positive of that .... The problem for me is that he tried and he helped try to break up this country and that's what I'm dead set against. Where the hell are we going bringing in people like that here to cause more trouble?" O'Dwyer was described as born and raised in Quebec, though not anti-French or anti-Quebec.

Inside the *Star* a story by Quebec's Denis Massicotte gives the perspective of a French-language editor and publisher:

> Joe McCarthy would be proud if he visited our nation's capital. If the devout members of the We-Love-Canada-So-Much crowd who are screaming for David Levine's head get their way, we will soon be able to ask people in important positions in Canada: "How did you ever get your job?" "I may not be qualified but I can swear that I'm not at this time and I have never been a member of a separatist organization" will become the answer of choice.
>
> The collective hysteria displayed by the Ottawa media is frightening on the eve of National Assembly discussions on the Calgary constitutional agreement .... The screams of horror from the nation's capital clash totally with the wonderful spirit of Calgary. For Ontario Premier Mike Harris to side with the angry mob shows the level of intolerance that truly exists.
>
> Jacques Parizeau once said he would be sure of a referendum win if he could get a second Brockville, a reference to the story about English Canadians stomping on the Quebec flag.

Le Journal de Montréal. In *Le Journal de Montréal* columnist Franco Nuovo, having noted the steadfastness of the Ottawa board, raises the question "If

David Levine was so very good and competent, why did Quebec let him slip away?" Lucien Bouchard and Bernard Landry spoke with verve and passion about Mr. Levine's merits. Even the National Assembly threw him a bouquet. Why then wasn't he chosen to head up the CHUM (Centre Hospitalier de l'Université de Montréal), the amalgamated hospital formed from Notre-Dame, Hôtel-Dieu, and Saint-Luc?

Specialists advised that Levine was the right man for the CHUM job, writes Nuovo. But because he was too identified with the Notre-Dame he was pushed aside. Nuovo notes that the person who did get the job, Cécile Cléroux, had no experience, and the result has been a bit of a mess. Why was the Wayne Gretzky of hospital administration discharged in favour of a peewee, he asks. Maybe it was due to technocratic or political stupidity. He leaves the reader only with questions, no answers.

Le Journal de Montréal has two other stories: one about the National Assembly vote denouncing intolerance towards Levine; the other a report on what union leader Jocelyne Fortier thought of Levine, whom she knew well. According to Fortier, Levine was known "for his very human approach, his respect for the employees, his careful listening and his openness of mind."

Columnist Michel Auger faults Prime Minister Jean Chrétien for being slow to defend David Levine's constitutional rights. Mr. Chrétien refused to say that sovereignty is a legitimate political option and that those who promote it are not traitors but citizens participating in a political debate, a right granted by the constitution, writes Auger. When Chrétien says "no other country in the world would be as tolerant to sovereignists," we don't know whether to take it as a praise of Canadian tolerance or a thinly veiled threat. The same ambiguity is expressed by the Plan B[7] and the attempt to have moves to achieve sovereignty declared illegal, and, eventually, treasonous. Some Ottawa citizens already perceive it as such.

Auger also discusses Brian Mulroney's policy of "national reconciliation," which reasoned that change would not come by excluding sovereignists from the life of the nation. Liberal MP Mauril Bélanger made the same point when he said that we should not be surprised if Quebecers were to separate if we spend our time excluding them. So under Mulroney we saw former péquistes Yves Duhaime and Denis de Belleval named to important positions in the federal administration without passing a loyalty test, since the government considered them legitimate. "Opposed to their own, but legitimate." Auger suggests asking whether the Chrétien government has appointed any known separatist to the federal public service, even aside from the politically sensitive jobs for which they might seem to be inappropriate. By contrast, the Canadian government saw nothing remarkable, a few months ago, when the Canadian ambassador in Paris gave a round of lectures in Quebec to promote Canadian unity. He saw no conflict with the neutrality called for in his position.

Under such circumstances, Auger concludes that the Prime Minister gives the impression of encouraging a continuation of what happened in Ottawa, as did Stéphane Dion when he described the scene as ugly and unacceptable but said he was ready to "explain" the feelings of those opposed to Levine's nomination.

There is an enormous gulf in understanding between the *Ottawa Citizen*, the *Ottawa Sun* and CFRA's Lowell Green on the one side, and *Le Devoir*, *Le Journal de Montréal* and *Le Droit* on the other, with exceptions being made for certain individuals within those institutions. Each side seems to consider the position of the other so unreasonable as not to be taken seriously. The latter group argues, "So what if he's a separatist?" The former argues, "Separatism may not be legally treason, but it is morally repugnant, and taxpayers of Ontario should not have to reward or otherwise encourage it." Bridging the chasm means looking at the reality of many francophones who dither over a separatist option. Many have positive feelings towards Canada, but also towards Quebec, with which they identify more closely for reasons of language and culture. Their aim is not to harm Canada, but to find a better place for themselves. That is why the "Lamb Lobby" may have the right idea after all; the more hostile the reaction from the rest of Canada, the more likely the chances of the negative attitude towards separatism becoming a self-fulfilling prophecy. By contrast, as some letter-writers have indicated, a friendly, understanding approach will encourage people to seek solutions within the existing basic constitutional framework. This is not to say that Quebec anglophones don't have legitimate grievances. But it is hard to see how rescinding Levine's appointment and dismissing the hospital board would have achieved a positive outcome.

NOTES

1. Gratton was also among those who spoke at the May 19 meeting. He told me in an interview that he had hoped his letter, faxed the previous week, would have been published earlier, in time to be read before the meeting.
2. The English presented here is a translation from *Le Devoir's* French, which is not entirely accurate, if the *Citizen* correctly quotes Harris today. See the *Citizen's* version later in this chapter.
3. The reference is to Copps's budget, as Canadian Heritage Minister, of some $20 million for flag production and distribution.
4. No French accents appeared in the *Free Press* story.
5. In the days ahead, people questioned whether Chrétien applied this principle in appointing people to the Senate.
6. His letter might be compared with that of Dr. Norman Levine, May 20.
7. Plan B is the term used to describe the federal government's hard-line strategy, since 1993, for dealing with separatism, as opposed to Plan A, which refers to a softer, more conciliatory approach. Intergovernmental Affairs minister Stéphane Dion is generally associated with Plan B. (See, among many references, "Plan B is dead, senator claims," The Montreal *Gazette,* March 28, 1998.)

CHAPTER FOUR

REAliGNMENT of AttiTUdEs, MAy 22 ANd AfTER

The decision of the Ottawa Hospital Board to stand by its appointment of David Levine was a landmark in the shifting media coverage and changing public opinion. The build-up of pressure to force Levine's resignation was partly fuelled by the hope and expectation that the board would bow to the fiercely negative commentary appearing in the media. Since the board made its decision, however, interest in the story declined and a sizable part of the opposition, having decided that further protest would be pointless, sought more constructive action in the interests of a workable health system in Ottawa.

Nevertheless, as of July 1998, a determined minority still keep up their opposition by picketing businesses owned by board members. This group, admonished in articulate letters to the *Citizen*, appears to have gained little public sympathy. The *Sun's* Earl McRae continues to urge the troops to keep up the fight but support seems to be steadily eroding, judging from the overall tone and volume of commentary and letters in the press.

The board's decision was also a turning point for the French-language media. If Levine had been fired, it would have enormously fortified the separatist cause in Quebec. Once the decision to retain Levine was made and news stories about it were published on Friday May 22 and the weekend, the French media, with the exception of *Le Droit,* allowed the issue to fade. Sustained scrutiny of parallels between the fate of separatists in the rest of Canada and federalists in the PQ government might not always be to Quebec's advantage, as Dr. Augustin Roy argued in a letter to *Le Devoir* May 26, published June 3. Roy challenged: "Find me members of the upper echelon Quebec public service and its different bodies who are not separatists! Caisse de dépôt et de placement, Office de la langue Française, Société des alcools, Hydro-Québec ...." Levine's own New York job of delegate general was opened up by the departure of a Liberal appointee, who anticipated that acceptance of separatism would be an essential requirement under the PQ. As a lesson in anglo intolerance outside Quebec, contrasting with Quebec's supposedly greater tolerance of minorities, the Levine case no longer served as a clear-cut, stellar example. After all, Levine did keep his job.

The situation in which the newspaper *Le Droit* finds itself is noticeably different from that of the other French media. It is concerned that the backlash against the Levine appointment will undercut concessions made regarding the Montfort Hospital and the availability of health services in the French language. For *Le Droit* continuing vigilance is necessary. The Levine case and fallout were tracked carefully during the summer months.

Saturday, May 23

Toronto Star. The *Toronto Star* provides major coverage on the Levine affair, which had, until May 22, been treated as a relatively minor event. William Walker's front-page, banner headline reads "Why ugly unity fight exploded in Ottawa": "This city, a capital often derided as the quiet grey epitome of Canadian federalism, bared its fangs this week and the effects may linger for a long time," he continues.

Walker parallels the Levine affair to the 1989 desecration of the Quebec flag in Brockville, and describes the hostile radio and newspaper reaction to Levine as a "surprise gift—value to be determined—to sovereignist forces in Quebec." Walker quotes pollster Frank Graves of Ekos Research Associates as saying that the intemperate language and cancellation of hospital donations totalling more than $1 million could "certainly" have a potential impact on Quebec sovereignty, particularly in the short term: "if this had come in the middle of a referendum or an election campaign, it could have been disastrous."

Ottawa Regional Councillor Alex Munter is quoted as saying he was embarrassed at the image of the city displayed on the national stage: "This has become much more than an issue about the hiring of a hospital administrator. It's an issue about whether there's hope for this country and whether we can get along. If we can't get along in the national capital, what does that say for the country?" Former Ottawa Mayor Marion Dewar is also reported to have called the two Ottawa right-wing newspapers "irresponsible" and incendiary in their handling of the issue.

CFRA talk-show host Lowell Green, also interviewed for Walker's story, claims that if Levine were appointed president and CEO "it will destroy this community": Ottawa taxpayers are helpless against the federal government's hiring of separatists and now "finally here's a chance where we get a little even. Here's our chance to say No."

Sandro Contenta writes an interesting and illuminating story on how separatist-federalist feelings are kept in check in Quebec ("Quebecers graced by indifference," A27). He interviewed people in a community where francophones and anglophones live next door to each other, noting that they just ignore politics and keep their tempers in check: "Quebecers have learned to live, work and play with their political opponents," he writes. "We're too evenly divided to do that sort of thing," McGill philosopher Charles Taylor is quoted as saying: "When your neighbour and your brother-in-law uphold a different political option, it leads to much greater tolerance. Otherwise, we would have destroyed ourselves."

Contenta provides some important details about Quebec hiring practices that are useful in combatting prejudice. Although the PQ replaced some of their foreign trade representatives who were not sovereignists, they also appointed Charles Lapointe, a federal cabinet minister under Pierre Trudeau, to a top job in the tourism sector, and "Guy Coulombe, the top civil servant in Liberal premier Robert Bourassa's government, was named head of the provincial police force."

Contenta notes that well-known federalists Keith Henderson, leader of the Equality Party, and William Johnson, now leader of Alliance Quebec, both support the decision to give Levine the job. In Johnson's view, "The man should be judged on his competence and he clearly was deemed competent so he should be hired and he should be retained. So clearly, justice was done." Johnson also notes that the sovereignist movement is seen as perfectly legitimate in Quebec. As for Premier Harris's statement that he would have preferred giving the job to a foreigner rather than a Quebec separatist, Johnson commented: "The premier made an ass of himself." Charles Taylor also viewed as unacceptable Premier Harris's dismissal of freedom of opinion guaranteed by the Charter of Rights and Freedoms: "Someone like that in an important public office in Canada, who says something that seems to invite people to ignore the Charter, ought to recant or resign. This is not what we elect people to do."

The *Star* also editorializes on the same subject, arguing that Levine should be given a chance to get on with the job, and that he would have to work hard to gain public trust ("Separatist witch hunt"). Gordon Guyatt of the Medical Reform Group is quoted approvingly, "This is an issue of political freedom in a democratic society." The editorial concludes: "If it's okay to blacklist a separatist candidate, why not a Commie? Or a Green candidate? Or maybe a New Democrat. Or a Family Coalition candidate. Or a Libertarian. There's no end to it. And the next target might be you or me."

Finally, the *Star's* national affairs columnist, Rosemary Speirs, attacks Premier Mike Harris ("Mike Harris needs lesson on human rights law," E5) who "might have the mob on his side when he says he wouldn't have hired a separatist to head a big public institution in his province. But he doesn't have Canadian law on his side." Speirs notes that the Ontario Human Rights Code forbids discrimination in accommodation or employment and recognizes the equal and unalienable rights of all people in accord with the United Nations' Universal Declaration of Human Rights, which contains a specific section on political freedom. As Premier, Harris had the duty to reflect the spirit of the Ontario code when speaking out on human rights issues, writes Speirs: "The fact that he may find the PQ separatist agenda repulsive doesn't justify discrimination against any of its adherents, any more than against, say, a member of the Liberal party or the NDP."

Montreal *Gazette*. The Montreal *Gazette* devotes most of the front page of its Review section to the Levine affair with a 6 inch by 9 inch photo of a smiling, open-shirted Levine carrying a garment bag over his arm. Inside is Don Macpherson's column which suggests that if Levine were really such a dedicated separatist, the best thing he could have done to help the movement would have been to resign, claim discrimination and thus become a martyr for the cause. The only chance for the separatists, now that he has been retained, is a continued battle with anti-separatist protesters. Otherwise the issue will be a "one-week wonder," at least from a national perspective.

Josh Freed's column on page 2 of the *Gazette's* first section provides a most insightful portrait of David Levine, written from personal knowledge of the man that was acquired long before the present incident. For one thing, the picture of him as a diehard separatist gives way to disillusionment with the PQ's shift to the right after the first referendum. He "turned in his card in 1981." But as Levine was on a first-name basis with several cabinet ministers, they came to his help when he was denied a chance to head up the mega Centre Hospitalier Université and offered him the New York job. Freed says:

> [I have] debated Quebec politics with Levine several times in recent years, and frankly I'd say he was as critical of the PQ as I am. He was disillusioned with their move away from social democracy and their cuts in medicine and other social areas. He didn't see the real point of independence any more, which he thought could strengthen Quebec's vulnerability to the United States.

His real interest, according to Freed, is hospital administration; hence his application for the Ottawa job. "Frankly," says Freed, "I suspect Levine could have told the howling Ottawa press that he was no longer a great fan of sovereignty or the PQ government. But he behaved honorably and refused to knuckle under to the McCarthy-style pressure. In the end he got the job anyway, but the episode leaves scars."

Freed made a number of observations about politicians and the media:

> The Ontario crowd that attacked him doesn't disturb me—you can find excitable crowds everywhere. But the mayor of Ottawa and the premier of Ontario should both be forced to come to Montreal for a two-week remedial seminar in tolerance training .… Another group that might consider joining the seminar is the local Ottawa press corps that spent weeks fanning the flames for this witch hunt. This week, an *Ottawa Citizen* editorial suggested that the issue was no longer whether or not Levine was once a PQ candidate. The real issue was that he had become too controversial to do a good job. They didn't mention that story by story the Ottawa media helped feed the rage that created the "controversy."

In the end, if you really want to ban everyone who ever worked for the PQ from holding a good job in Canada, then the logical extension is to declare the PQ an illegal party. We should just forbid the PQ from running in elections, force it underground and tell those who belong to it to find other ways to achieve their goals—rallies, protests and if need be, bullets and bombs. But you might end up living someplace that reminds you more of Algeria than Canada.

Well said, Mr. Freed. Anyone hostile to Levine should read this column.

Ottawa Citizen. The *Ottawa Citizen's* news coverage is favourable to Levine. The front-page headline gives his perspective: "'Calm down,' Levine pleads," and the subhead presents a concerned and active new administrator, "New hospital chief starts job early to try to quell tensions." By engaging in the job ahead of time, Levine reinforces the notion that further resistance is futile.

Jack Aubry begins his story:

David Levine, the region's controversial new hospital czar, says he wants to help "calm down" his opponents by leaving his job as the representative of Quebec earlier than planned. He will take on his new duties June 15, six weeks earlier than originally scheduled.

Levine is then quoted as saying that the board had done the right thing in apologizing to the community for not having anticipated the tension produced by his appointment.

The story does not eliminate the negative feelings that may linger among federalists: Aubry notes that Levine is unwilling to dissociate himself from his separatist past and that there is an absence of Canadian symbols in his New York office, where the interview took place:

The uproar over Mr. Levine's hiring … has developed into a national unity crisis. An attempt to defuse the controversy in a press conference last week failed when he refused to disclose his position on unity …. Although the office is listed in the New York yellow pages under "Canada," a geographically challenged American visitor would be hard pressed to find out which country the province is part of by dropping in on Mr. Levine's workplace.

The story also quotes New York investment bankers as saying that Levine came across as low-key on separatism.

Ottawa Sun. The *Ottawa Sun* gives extensive coverage with two columns, a news story and a cartoon. Earl McRae's column lampoons David Levine's skills—if they were all that essential, he says, the health of the region would hinge upon his continued well-being; hence the headline, "Say a prayer for Levine's health." Obviously, since this is not the case, then denying Levine his job can hardly be catastrophic. McRae contrasts the Levine hiring with elections in the Southern U.S.: unlike the racist Alabama governor, elected by racist seg-regationists, "David Levine was *not* elected. He was appointed. By 32 people. Who are also not elected, but appointed. By a tiny group of unaccountable elit-ists. The people had no say. They would not have elected Levine. There's the difference." McRae may be right, but he has no just claim to certainty about this. The people who have heard only about Levine's separatism are naturally op-posed; those who hear of his good qualities tend to change their minds.

Stephanie Rubec's news story gives important coverage of the reaction in Quebec to the May 19 meeting. The article is headed "Levine furor gives jolt to federalism," and she opens with "Outaouais unity groups believe the contro-versy surrounding David Levine has dealt a small blow to the federal cause." The story quotes a spokesperson for the federalist group Solidarité Outaouais Solidarity as saying that comments at the May 19 meeting probably sent some Quebecers towards the sovereignist camp, but that it is important to the group that Quebecers understand the anger as directed towards separatists, not Quebecers as such. An English rights group, Outaouais Alliance, expressed concern that David Levine's political views be kept under wraps in his new job. The story also quotes Prime Minister Jean Chrétien's statement about the lack of outcry in Quebec when federalists lost their jobs in a PQ takeover. Former Mayor Marion Dewar is reported as saying that people are under the false impression that they will not be able to get hospital service in English: "They're angry and hurt and frightful and they have to take it out on somebody so it all came out."

Alan Fotheringham's column, "No more country, no more job," which also appeared in the *Financial Post*, labels the pro-Levine forces as "politi-cally correct." The CBC, as a counterweight to the other local media at the height of the anti-Levine coverage, also came under fire by Fotheringham: "The earnestly correct anchorpersons on the CBC have been earnestly seeking out every usual suspect on the empathetic side who can emote that this poor chap should not be deprived [of] his job because of his 'political' beliefs." He trots out the old joke about the lifeguard who couldn't swim but got the job because he was bilingual, and says it's wrong that Levine, not believing in Canada, should be rewarded with a $300,000 job. Clearly the "gut and feeling" across Canada for keeping this country together was just not understood in Ottawa.

Fotheringham concludes: "Despite the stubborn and nervous vote of the board on confirmation this week, he will be gone. Trust me."[1] Those words may come home to haunt him.

Two letters on Levine were also published. One, from Leonard Belaire,

104 THE DAVID LEVINE AFFAIR

extolled the merits of genuine patriotism without drawing explicit conclusions relating to Levine. In the second letter, R. Martinelli, proclaims himself an anti-separatist, but is in favour of giving Levine a chance to do the job for which he was hired:

> I do not believe for one bit, as some may think, that an anglophone patient will not be able to get service in English. I also doubt that bilingualism will be the only factor among other skills considered when (or if) staff cuts are required in the hospital.

Martinelli allowed, though, that the selection process might have been flawed.

Finally, the *Sun's* cartoon provides a bit of comic relief, showing an elderly couple watching TV: "Now that the *Hospital Fight* is over, I can get back to the *Hockey Fight.*"

Financial Post. A letter from an English-speaking resident of Dollard-des-Ormeaux opposes Arthur Drache's column of May 20 on the grounds that "thinking again" about (i.e., rescinding) the appointment of David Levine, because of his political beliefs, would be contrary to the Charter of Rights and Freedoms.

Winnipeg and Halifax Press. The *Winnipeg Free Press* carries an editorial in favour of Levine's appointment, judging him to be a careerist with limited loyalty to the PQ. Federalists should be "standing high on the battlements waving to the defecting separatists, inviting them to turn their coats and flee to safety in the federalist camp." The smart separatists would leave early to get the best jobs, claims the *Free Press.*

The Halifax *Chronicle Herald's* editorial "Separation hysteria" denounces the reaction to Levine's appointment in Ottawa:

> If David Levine had been named head of Canada's Armed Forces, then perhaps the hysteria surrounding his appointment would be justified. But he's just going to head the new amalgamated Ottawa Hospital. His separatist leanings would hardly seem to matter much in that context.

The editorial goes on to describe the uproar against Levine and takes a slap at Ontario Premier Mike Harris, accusing him of "pandering to … misplaced anti-separatist sentiment." After wondering whether we are going to "blacklist every Quebecer who ever had a separatist thought," the editorial concludes: "Reason will prevail. And that is why Canada is not a gulag, to borrow a phrase from the most famous separatist of them all. We can't let narrow-minded people turn it into one."

Le Devoir. *Le Devoir's* front-page column by Manon Cornellier ("The heavy challenge of Levine") argues that, in spite of many people who had turned against the May 19 mob, the remaining minority could still make David Levine's work difficult. The group "made such a clamour that it is now feared that francophones will pay the price," she writes.

One source of difficulty for the Ottawa Hospital board is the existence of informants in the amalgamated hospitals; one forced the board to announce Levine's appointment prematurely and another leaked the decision to keep David Levine, she reveals. (In the next chapter we explore circumstances relating to the announcement of Levine's appointment.) It is not clear whether this tactic was motivated by patent opposition to Quebec sovereignty or designed to exploit anti-francophone sentiment and spread irritation concerning separatism. Board members Agnès Jaouich and Lucien Bradet are quoted as saying that all hospital restructuring brings about strong resistance, but that an explosive mix developed when some individuals used the Levine nomination to stir up prejudice and latent fear. Several people at the Civic fear for their jobs, not being bilingual.

In Cornellier's view, Levine is a lightning rod in a rumbling thunderstorm, but no one believed the tumult would reach the dimensions it had. David Levine's nomination ought not to be opposed, given his abilities. But, in light of the harm done, Levine will be closely watched by a vengeful minority for whom respect for fundamental rights depends on one's political allegiance.

Also in *Le Devoir* a page-length column reviewing the English language press notes that the *Citizen* editorialists are harder on David Levine than columnist Randall Denley. Primary attention is given to the *Globe and Mail's* May 22 editorial, which again condemns the May 19 hostility to the Levine appointment. The *Globe* argued that reaction to the board's decision to keep Levine demonstrated that Quebec Vice-Premier Bernard Landry was wrong to say, earlier in the week, that the reaction was proof of the existence of two nations in the country— *"ours and theirs."*

Le Journal de Montréal. Pierre Bourgault, writing in *Le Journal de Montréal,* sees in David Levine's Quebec career proof of the province's openness to non-French ethnic groups, which is what sovereignists have been proclaiming for forty years: "Levine, Jew and anglophone, is 'pure wool' like all of us. That's what English Canada can't stand."

Bourgault takes a swipe at Prime Minister Jean Chrétien, calling him petty and crude for defending freedom of expression and at the same time haranguing the nasty separatists. Premier Harris comes in for special whipping: he "embodied perfectly the good old racist base of English Canada in asserting that he would prefer to choose a foreigner than a Québécois."

What Harris said was bad enough, but Bourgault misrepresents him and exaggerates the insult by replacing Harris's word, "separatist," with the word

"Québécois." Premier Harris would not have said that he prefers choosing a foreigner over a Québécois. It's true that Levine is a Québécois, but Harris is not against Levine for being Québécois; he is against him for being a separatist. Bourgault stirs up mischief and foments anti-anglo feelings among Quebecers, perhaps with a view to furthering separatism in Quebec. Such distortion of truth should be exposed. Bourgault's claim that Harris "has placed himself on the side of hatred and intolerance from the height of his position as Premier of Ontario" is more credible.

Bourgault chastizes English Canadian journalists who have done everything, for three years, to stir up hatred and contempt for Quebecers. "Shame to the newspapers which published letters calling for 'the punishment for traitors' for Levine." Shame on the *Ottawa Sun* columnist who wrote that "There are circumstances where the interests of the nation justify civil disobedience." Triple shame on the *Financial Post* columnists who asserted that "intolerance is justified when it is a matter of combatting a harm comparable to apartheid or the laws of Hitler." And shame on English Canadian intellectuals: "Apart from certain exceptions, they are conspicuous by their absence. They lay low and keep quiet. Guilty of abstention."

In his *Le Journal de Montréal* political column, Jules Richer analyses the reaction of Ottawa's English-language media to the board's reaffirmation of the David Levine appointment. In Richer's view the media were as unchanged and inflammatory as ever, particularly the *Ottawa Sun* editorial and the *Citizen's* column by John Robson. But the *Citizen's* "So, David Levine stays—and damn the consequences" is a shade different from the *Sun's* "Levine must go!" in my reading. The *Citizen* at least accepts the reality of Levine staying, even though the editorial claims that the issue will fester for months or years.

Richer seems to me wrong to suppose that there is no change in the *Citizen*. John Robson's column is not an adequate expression of the newspaper's stance. To justify his thesis, perhaps, Richer promoted Robson to "head of the editorial section," but Robson's actual title is deputy editorial pages editor, second in command of the editorial pages. Robson's style is dry, making his readership likely limited, but he raises a reasonable question, picked up by Richer, about how Quebecers would react to the nomination of a partitionist at the head of a hospital in their own province.

More importantly, Richer restricts his concern to individual commentators and pays no attention to the significant change in tone brought about by Daniel Leblanc's front-page article headed "Levine was once a Liberal, too" and by the sympathetic Levine biography on page A3. Richer's impressions about the newspaper are misleading.

Richer also reviews the comments of radio phone-in callers to CFRA Radio. Bernie in Ottawa said that the battle against Levine "was not yet over" and was very worried about the future of anglophones who were employed in the amalgamated hospital. Another listener, Marion, denounced Quebec Liberal leader Jean Charest's defence of Levine, asking what he had done to save the anglophone hospital in his own Sherbrooke constituency when it was closed down. "Nothing," she said. Finally Heidi, who said she had known the horrors of the Holocaust, held that "various things happening in Quebec show similarities to the Nazi regime at its beginnings." For her, the charisma of Lucien Bouchard resembled that of Adolf Hitler and she feared that Ontario would undergo his influence.

Sunday, May 24

Ottawa Citizen. The *Citizen* gives the Levine issue a respite in its news and columns, but carries twelve letters under the neutral heading "Levine decision: Relief or an insult?" Sheryl Bartlett of Kanata is relieved at the reaffirmation of Levine's appointment. Michael Valentine of Ottawa thinks that it would have been unconscionable for the board to do otherwise and that withdrawing support will hurt only the future patients of the hospital, not the board or CEO. Scott Fairless says that Levine was a wise choice and that the residents of Ottawa-Carleton owed him an apology: "Nowhere is there any evidence that Mr. Levine has allowed his political views to influence his previous positions as health-care administrator. Separatism is far less of a threat to the nation's well-being than ideological intolerance."

A letter by Keith Christopher of Nepean repeats the familiar charge that melding of French and English cultures is not achievable by a separatist. Paul Robertson Day of Kanata writes a tongue-in-cheek letter saying that the revelation that Levine was once Liberal made him withdraw his support: "Do we really want someone associated with a party famous for its arrogance and do-whatever-it-takes-to-get-elected mentality to be running the Ottawa Hospital?" he asks. Mark Lane of Ottawa views the board's apology as hypocritical; if they were really sorry about the fuss they caused they would have fired David Levine, he writes. Albert Tunis of Ottawa congratulates the board for "standing firm in the face of invective and insult of an emotional, irrational outburst from the media and a segment of the public." Walter Thomson of L'Orignal opposes giving a position of high honour to a separatist.

James Steen of Ottawa looks at the credentials of those characterized as "bigots" by the pro-Levine side, and finds them admirable: Second World War veterans; unilingual English nurses; doctors; people who wondered why the Grace and Riverside hospitals were closed and the world-renowned Civic reduced to a community hospital; all those who thought "board member Pierre de Blois was arrogant when he said anyone who spoke against Mr. Levine's appointment was ill-informed"; elderly people who think fundraising will be made difficult; and finally, "all those who think public boards should be accountable to the communities they serve."

Jake Drupsteen ridicules Prime Minister Jean Chrétien's May 21 claim in the *Citizen* that "In Canada political considerations are not a question that we ask for employment, we look at the qualities of the person to serve." Comments Drupsteen acidly: "We can now look forward at long last to the end of patronage appointments to plum government jobs. In future, appointments will be based on qualifications rather than political affiliation. Imagine, a former Reform MP being appointed to the Senate instead of a tired Liberal!"

Dale Hibbard of Aylmer, a retired journalist, takes the *Ottawa Citizen* severely to task for its handling of the Levine affair. He accuses the newspaper of "blunderingly condoning coercion" by "editorially aligning itself with inquisitional fanatics. He also denounces the use of the word "traitor" to describe Levine in a May 14 front-page story, calling it a "broadsheet indecency that would make any reasonably educated, reasonably intelligent and reasonably cultured Canadian uncontrollably throw up." The *Citizen* "has gone off the deep end. The publisher, Russell Mills, should have the spunk to say so."

Robert Sauvé of Ottawa describes himself as part of the May 19 "unruly mob" that sang "O Canada" and called for the firing of David Levine and the trustees. Though not comfortable with the anti-French comments, he held his nose and "shouted with the best of them because I am fed up" with, among other things, "officials who arrogantly treat the legitimate concerns of the people as the inconvenient braying of uninformed dolts."

A final letter, spread across four columns at the bottom of the page, is strongly in favour of Levine ("Levine soon demonstrated his competence, improved his French in Verdun"). The letter is signed "Dr. André Bourque, Head, Family Medicine Department, Centre Hospitalier Angrignon, Verdun." It reveals that after Levine became executive director of the Verdun General Hospital, where there was a strong francophone and Catholic tradition, there was some expression of religious, ethnic or political intolerance. "In a very short time, he demonstrated his competence and was in command. Mr. Levine met no form of discrimination related to his religious, ethnic or political background during his 10 years at Verdun .... He proved to be a rather extraordinary hospital administrator ... and his French improved immensely," writes Dr. Bourque.

Ottawa Sun. The *Ottawa Sun* pursues the subject with renewed vigour in its opinion columns especially. Ottawa Mayor Jim Watson, having earlier provided support to the anti-Levine cause, throws his weight behind the effort to leave the divisiveness behind and cooperate with those in charge of the new hospital. In a page-five news story headed "Mayor says fights bleed hospital," Jacki Leroux writes, "Ottawa Mayor Jim Watson has three words for federalists still trying to fight David Levine as the new CEO of the Ottawa Hospital: Get over it. 'The board has made its decision and we should move on,' he said yesterday." Mayor Watson supports the idea of a more accountable board, but adds that it is "not really fair" that the board is vulnerable to criticism since most of the members are volunteers.

A humour column by Ron Corbett, "Final bons mots on David Levine," indicates that tensions are now easing, for many people, on the whole affair. He wonders how much it would cost to get rid of all separatists if getting rid of just one of them would cost over $200,000.

Douglas Fisher revisits the Levine issue in a *Sun* column headed "On the road to separation," a very insightful study about the tensions in Ottawa and Canada generally regarding the future of Quebec. Fisher notes that when, in an earlier column, he supported the French-language Montfort Hospital based on his experience as a patient there, he got "more nasty or derisive needling than from any other column published here in the last decade."

He thinks the Levine affair might have been anticipated, in light of "clear signals, locally and nationally, of the widening, deepening anger among English-speaking Canadians at the PQ, the BQ, and the long-fermenting issue of Quebecois intentions to separate and split Canada physically and constitutionally." A large proportion of people want no more concessions to Quebec, he writes, "no more pussyfooting and 'bonne ententism.'" As Fisher sees it, the feelings were reflected in the hard line taken by Intergovernmental Affairs Minister Stéphane Dion with the so-called "Plan B." Contributing to the angry feelings were tales about "billions blown on official bilingualism and its ruination of the federal bureaucracy and the armed services. Equity and fairness in federal pay and promotions are gone."

Exposure of these anti-French feelings at the May 19 meeting received a lot of attention in Quebec and would likely turn undecided Quebecers more towards the separatist option, Fisher felt, echoing Chantal Hébert of *La Presse*. Revelation of the anglo animosity might well prove a federalist disaster. Fisher claims there may be an even higher proportion of people in the rest of Canada than in Quebec who would like to see Quebec separate. Fisher concludes: "The Levine case is an indicator of a widespread readiness on the anglo side of the duality, and at least a forecast there can be no sweetheart deal or an eventual spirit of co-operation and camaraderie if the one country becomes two."

Fisher's claims about the anglo mood were somewhat confirmed by my own unscientific sampling of letter writers whom I interviewed. In some cases, their views seemed poorly thought out. For instance, some treated as "traitors" those who advocated separatism, but agreed on questioning that a separate Quebec would be preferable to bilingualism imposed elsewhere in Canada. Behind this apparent inconsistency lies the logic of frustration: both parties agree that when a relationship sours, splitting may be the least worse option, and then one blames the other for the break-up. We will return to this question in the next chapter.

Christina Blizzard, the *Sun's* Queen's Park columnist, takes the peculiar position that David Levine should not resign but that the board that hired him should. Then, faced with a new board, David Levine would see he no longer had their confidence and "it should follow that he will simply resign." Firing Levine would be wrong because, she writes, "Much as you and I may find

Levine's politics repulsive, he has a right to his views and, having been given the job he shouldn't be fired for his political beliefs." What drives this thinking is partly her expressed belief that David Levine will have the power to increase the number of separatists who work in Ottawa hospitals while laying off federalist supporters. "I'm not saying he would," she cautions, "But that's the kind of can of worms you're opening here." She concludes with a round defence of freedom of opinion: "Remember this, though: Separatism is a doctrine based on xenophobia and racism. But no matter how much we are repelled by Levine's politics, he has a right to his beliefs. If we demand our politicians fire him, aren't we being racist and xenophobic also?" Blizzard's high tone about respecting freedom of belief is hard to square with her devious plan to force Levine to resign. Don't fire him, but fix it so that he has to quit.

Michael Harris, the *Ottawa Sun's* national affairs columnist, castigates the board that appointed David Levine:

> At a time when French/English emotions are running high over the service cuts at the region's only French-language hospital, the Montfort, they have imported a separatist to build bridges between the two solitudes, which must now share reduced hospital services. It is an appointment that paves the way for Ernst Zundel to be named chairman of the Human Rights Commission. Outrage in hot pursuit of farce.

Harris follows this remark with an intemperate, unfair and deceptive claim: "Given that the party of David Levine builds bridges to its fellow Canadians with dynamite, it would be hard to invent a less fit candidate for the job, even after a good guzzle of Jack Daniels and a feed of magic mushrooms." Harris here seems to be fusing the PQ with the FLQ, a move which is patently unfair and, in my view, libelous if we take the "dynamite" as a reference to FLQ bombings.

The burden of Harris's argument in "Mulder & Co. prescribe poison pill," is that "the uproar created by [Levine's] appointment was inevitable," and that the hospital board should have avoided it by picking someone not affiliated with the PQ. Separatist beliefs are a disqualification, in Harris's mind, for "one of the plummiest jobs in the country they [the separatists] can't wait to leave." In answer to Pierre Bourgault's claim in *Le Journal de Montréal* that "[English Canada's] virulent racism is leading straight to war," Harris answers that the Quebec civil service is 99 percent francophone while minorities make up 20 percent of Quebec's population. The strident tone of Harris's article contrasts with the attempts by Mayor Jim Watson (mentioned in the previous chapter) to lower the heat in the public debate and come to terms with the new situation. Words like "bone-headed," "chicken-hearted," "witless squeal," and the like pepper Harris's column and fuel existing indignation.

Finally, in a letter about the Quebec legislature's motion denouncing intolerance towards David Levine, Frank Simek writes with heavy irony and some nice alliteration: "This is a well deserved lecture from the cherubs who chased hundreds of thousands of Canadians from la Belle Province by their tolerance. This is a rightful rebuke from the fearless defenders of individual freedoms armed with rulers to measure the size of alien letters in the shop windows. This is a wake-up call from the ultimate democrats who refuse to accept the result of any and all referenda unless it agrees with their gospel."

Le Journal de Montréal. Of the two *Journal* news stories pertaining to Levine, the first was simply a report on his Thursday meeting with the press in New York, calling for calm and saying that neither he nor the board had anticipated the furore, but that the board was handling things well.

The other story, by Gilles Pilon, adds a new and useful bit of information to David Levine's biographical dossier. In a light-hearted vein, and parenthetically, Jacques Parizeau, former head of the PQ, told a group of about 700 sovereignists that not everything had been told about David Levine. Not wanting to add to Levine's miseries during the fray, Mr. Parizeau felt he could now say that Levine had been one of his MBA students at the École des Hautes Études Commerciales. "Mr. Levine was a brilliant student, but he asked me if he might write his first examination in English, promising me to do the subsequent ones in French, which he did," said Parizeau, adding that Levine ended his studies with the top mark in his class.

Monday, May 25
Ottawa Sun. The *Ottawa Sun* keeps up the interest with three columnists and one letter-writer expressing divided opinions. Only Earl McRae maintains an unabated push for action against Levine.

Linda Williamson's column analyses coverage of Levine's appointment. She states that "honest opposition to Levine's appointment" was being described as "an intolerable, hysterical, McCarthyist witch-hunt" in the *Gazette.* What was not getting attention, she claimed, was the dismay felt by those who suddenly

> found themselves being branded McCarthyites, bigots and worse (yes, that would include the *Sun* and other papers)—simply because they dared suggest that someone who has worked for the breakup of Canada might not be the best person to head a newly amalgamated bilingual hospital in the nation's capital.

Her way of putting it rather understates the position of many who opposed Levine. They did not just say he might not be the best person; they wanted to force his resignation. But her point remains that if one claims that political beliefs should be irrelevant to the kind of job Levine was offered, and that taking them into account would amount to McCarthyism, then the charge should apply even when decision-making is affected only in a minor way. Clearly, she and many others hold that there are cases where political beliefs do make some difference to suitability and that the charge of McCarthyism is misplaced in such cases.

Williamson is also critical of the way separatist commentators in Quebec seem to distort anti-separatist statements, making them appear more intolerant than they are and then denouncing them. "Agree with them and you're tolerant, but express an opinion and, strangely enough, you get accused of trying to repress free speech. Now, where's the dismay and outrage over that?" she concludes.

Ben Raynor, a federalist, dissociates himself from the "flag-waving public rantfest at the Civic last Tuesday." He yearns for the old days of low-key nationalism in Canada:

> To be honest, I kind of preferred the days when we all hummed and hawed over what exactly it meant to be Canadian, ducked our heads and blushed at our American neighbours' overt, eagle-emblazoned displays of nationhood, and took a subtle, modest and again, stereotypically Canadian, pride in not being so brash.

Earl McRae continues the fight against Levine, beginning with critical remarks about Ottawa Mayor Jim Watson for his urging people to "move on." He describes the hospital board as an "intransigent, unaccountable, board of separatist appeasers" and a "band of buffoons." He taunts his readers with the suggestion that by inaction they might be "spinelessly folding up [their] passions."

> I have had more phone calls on this than on any column I've written. All anti-board and Levine. From doctors, nurses, educators, lawyers, francophone and anglophone, professionals, blue collar, all concerned Canadian federalists. These people are not—as the soft-bellied community appeasers are screeching—dumb, redneck, braying morons.

He concludes his column with a list of names, telephone numbers and fax numbers for each of the board members, and a reference to Jean Charest's statement that "Leadership should rise above public opinion" as "imbecilic," noting that Charest himself was elected by public opinion.

Bob O'Connor's letter expresses his regret at the decision of the board to go "against the majority of the people's wishes." The battle against Levine was anti-separatist, not anti-French, and there was a united effort by French and English to say something to the separatists, he says. Now it is time to build a hospital: "I am a Canadian and as a Canadian I will now support the rebuilding of the hospital because the people of Ottawa-Hull and the area are more important than David Levine or his politics."

Ottawa Citizen. The paper publishes my article on the Levine issue, "When shouting 'McCarthyism' is 'McCarthyism'." It is a defence of the aptness of the "McCarthyism" tag in relation to the heated opposition to Levine and an answer to Earl McRae's objection to the use of the term.

Tuesday, May 26

Ottawa Sun. Once again David Levine is front-page material in the *Ottawa Sun* as a result of his appearance in Ottawa on May 25 for a press conference. A 6 inch by 9 inch picture of Levine, in a suit and tie, looking down, hand slightly outstretched and looking unusually large, takes up nearly half the page with a small inset headline "Outcry stuns Levine." By coincidence, perhaps, there is a scary headline accompanying the picture. In one-and-a-quarter inch type the headline reads, in four lines "Board axes 500 jobs." Anyone seeing the picture of Levine and the reference to the Board would likely conclude that Levine was already doing dirty work at the Ottawa Hospital. No doubt the juxtaposition would lead many nervous as well as curious individuals to buy the paper. It turns out, though, that the headline refers to trustees trimming $30 million in giving their okay to a $512 million school budget. The subheadline says as much, but in quarter-inch type.

Inside, Ron Corbett's column describes David Levine in a friendly vein: "Get to know me" was Levine's message. Corbett gives his personal reaction, which is that "Levine is even more of a careerist than I first suspected."

A news story by Andrew Matte reports Levine's surprise at the initial opposition that his appointment generated and his understanding of the strong emotions underneath. There were many issues, he said. "[Restructuring] in and of itself is a hard process for a community," he is reported as saying. "There is a desire to express a certain frustration about that. I was the lighting rod for a lot of that frustration which I hope over time I am going to be able to dispel." The story quotes Jack Kitts, head of anaesthesia at the hospital, as being impressed with Levine's credentials and abilities. Linda Schumacher, vice-president of nursing at the Riverside hospital site, agrees that Levine appears to be "an ideal CEO." Regular protester Nicholas Patterson, who was at the press conference, was reported as saying that "People should go to every board meeting and raise hell."

The *Sun* also reports on the previous day's exchange in Parliament between Deputy Prime Minister Herb Gray and Bloc MP Michel Gauthier. Asked whether he agreed that the Levine affair was an attack against freedom of opinion analogous to the 1970 October Crisis, Gray responded, "I think most Canadians, including Quebecers, find deplorable the efforts of the leader of the Bloc

Quebecois to promote his option with the Levine case." The debate is not brought to any depth.

Columnist Michael Harris alludes to the same parliamentary exchange in a single paragraph denouncing Michel Gauthier. His point is embedded in a blanket of name-calling:

> This partisan nig-nog tried to turn the ludicrous case of separatist col-league David Levine, the new administrator of the Ottawa Hospital, into a test case for the Canadian Charter of Rights and Freedoms, but the constitution sucks, right Mikey? Mike Harris of Ontario has it right. It would have been better to appoint a foreigner to this $330,000-a-year plum job, than a guy dedicated to the destruction of the country.

Two letters complete the *Sun's* attention to the Levine issue. The first, by Dan McIntyre, throws back at the *Sun* its editorial claim that Levine's hiring would "linger like a festering wound for months, possibly years, etc." "If so," writes McIntyre, "it will be the fault of newspapers like yours and not the fault of fair-minded Ontarians and Canadians including many who opposed the Levine hiring. We all need the Ottawa Hospital and all of its dedicated staff of health care professionals and support workers."

Daniel Kinsella supports a previous writer, Raynald Adams, on the matter of the relevance of the Canadian Charter of Rights and Freedoms to protection of David Levine's hiring. "Much as it pains you, the Charter protects all Canadians, not only the ones that you happen to agree with. Yes, even those who choose not to keep their political convictions 'private' instead of 'public.'" He suggests that abandoning this principle could lead to leftists rejecting Reform, Tory or Liberal candidates for government jobs.

Le Droit. *Le Droit* gives full front-page coverage to the Levine press conference, with an 8 inch by 7 inch picture of a somewhat aggressive-looking Levine pointing a finger at a questioner. The headline reads "'Everything is already underway.'" The story presents a "calm, serene, smiling" Levine:

> Without showing for a single second that he was affected by the popular expression of hostility towards him or by the campaign for his dismissal by various media, Mr. Levine expressed confidence in his ability to win over those opposed to his nomination, notably donors who threatened to stop giving to the hospital.

Writer Isabelle Ducas also quotes Jack Kitts' and Linda Schumacher's favourable reactions, noting that Nicholas Patterson's was the "only discordant note" at the press conference.

Three lengthy letters are printed in *Le Droit*. One, by Théo Martin, gives a graphic description of the May 19 meeting and laments the "Fascism of Canadian nationalism." Martin specifically mentions Ontario Premier Mike Harris and CTV's Mike Duffy as carrying on an exaggerated attack against Quebec separatists, and sports commentator Don Cherry as promoting xenophobia. Martin thinks that Levine's superior abilities would lead to a better hospital with more lives saved; it would be a pity if lives were lost because a handful of people, lacking humility and compassion, did not like a hospital director to have freedom of opinion.

Pierre LeBlanc of Gloucester writes to congratulate MP Mauril Bélanger for speaking out against the angry crowd on May 19 but accuses him of having undergone something of a conversion on the road to Damascus. The letter claims that Bélanger contributed to the sociopolitical climate that helped feed the hysteria over Levine, citing his organization of the Montreal love-in of 1995, his encouragement of civil disobedience in relation to Quebec's referendum law, and his promise and failure to deliver Canadian Heritage money for the Montfort Hospital. Leblanc seems willing, as he put it, to swing an incense-pot on Bélanger's behalf but not to seek his canonization just yet.

In a third letter, Gérard Laurin, head of the Hull PQ, fears that despite the expression of support for Levine, and the affirmation of freedom of opinion, the Ottawa Hospital board's excuses presage a paralyzing self-censorship regarding possible services in French. Laurin saw Mauril Bélanger's support for David Levine as "nebulous" and comparable to the reluctant way one might support the rights of an ex-convict:

> Which of the media had reminded people, clearly and firmly, on the airwaves or in their pages, that the Parti Québécois is a perfectly legal, democratically elected party, which respects as well as anyone the rights of minorities and even the imposed Constitution? Who has called attention to the abusive and malevolent language used to designate Quebec adherents to sovereignty? On the contrary, all the elected officials, federal and provincial, quick to criticize the least action by Quebec, saw fit to keep quiet and allow this to go on.

Echoing Lise Bissonnette, whom he mentions by name, Laurin concludes that Canadians need to have a lofty idea of freedoms, and they need equally to learn to recognize and respect these freedoms:

> Recent events will at least have brought to light of day the fragility of our democratic values and the necessity of denouncing those of our leaders who do not respect or get others to respect the most elementary obligations in the Canadian Charter of Rights.

Le Devoir. *Le Devoir's* Manon Cornellier reports on the press conference, giving many details already described in the other coverage. He also quotes Prime Minister Jean Chrétien's reaffirmation, now back in Ottawa, of his view that political beliefs should not enter into consideration when hiring a person:

> I think the problem was settled with the decision [of the board]. We should move on to other things. Unfortunately, this kind of problem happens on both sides from time to time. If we could settle once and for all the question of independence we would not have these problems.

BQ leader Gilles Duceppe finds this response unacceptable, reports Cornellier. Duceppe interprets Chrétien's words to mean that "if we don't speak of sovereignty, the problems won't arise. In other words, full freedom of opinion so long as we think the way he does." The Bloc intended to present a special motion congratulating the hospital board and reiterating the support of the House for the freedom of opinion guarantee in the Canadian and Quebec Charters, but the required unanimous consent to introduce the motion was not forthcoming. Duceppe is quoted as saying that when democracy is in danger, it is time to stand up and say so, and not bend spinelessly to intolerance: "I think one must get up and state clearly what one thinks. It transcends party politics. It's a matter of democracy. I think this is a problem for Canada, this attitude. So we should support those who are standing up."

WEdNESdAy, MAy 27

Ottawa Sun. This day further indicates that the *Ottawa Sun* is giving up its attack on Levine. A news story by Andrew Matte reports that the "fundraising arm of Ottawa's Civic Hospital has given David Levine a vote of confidence." Only one person of about 150 present at the previous night's annual general meeting of the foundation voiced concern, namely Nicholas Patterson. Gilles Desroches, a financial contributor, responded, "I frankly don't care about his politics. I think we should let him move forward with the task ahead of him. Then we should judge him."

Even Earl McRae seems finally to accept the Levine appointment as settled. In his column he reminds readers that Levine was on record as stating that unilingual anglophone staff at the Ottawa Hospital would *not* be faced with job discrimination. He encourages those who still wanted to hold protest rallies, but explains that "ethically I can't—as you've asked—actively lead your mobilizations. If one or more of you want to take it on, call me. I'll publish your names as contacts."

Likewise, Douglas Fisher, who earlier claimed that Levine would go, "trust me," today writes as if Levine will likely stay and deals instead with the nature and depth of the feelings expressed during the controversy:

The spontaneous eruption of protest should be taken as a warning to political leaders and major interest groups. There is a widening frustration among millions outside of Quebec, and unless its generating factors are openly faced and discussed with candor an explosion of wrath could come and blow away the myth so carefully built and insisted upon [by high-minded people in the name of national unity].

Fisher argues that the examples of Lucien Bouchard and Marcel Chaput, a research scientist with the National Research Council, prove that separatists will advance their agenda in the federal government. The high-minded believe that Levine will leave separatist beliefs out of his new job, but Fisher tells us he thought the same of Bouchard and Chaput. Is Fisher generalizing too hastily?

The *Sun* prints two letters on Levine. The first, by J.A. Strachan of Perth, presupposes the inadvisability of the Levine appointment and argues that the decision is one more example of leaders in society being out of touch with the people they serve. Anyone who thinks that the new CEO of the Ottawa Hospital will be able to function effectively "is living in another world," Strachan writes.

The second letter, by Len Herman, questions Prime Minister Chrétien's claim that political beliefs should not be taken into account when hiring: "So, how many PC's, Reformers and NDPers has the PM appointed to the Senate? And how many Liberals did former PM Mulroney appoint to the Senate?"

Le Journal de Montréal. Le Journal runs a story by Michelle Coude-Lord on the poor management of the hospital formed from the amalgamation of Notre Dame, Hotel-Dieu, and Saint-Luc, the hospital that rejected David Levine.

Thursday, May 28

Le Devoir. Graham Fraser's open letter in *Le Devoir* ("Lettre à David Levine") contrasts a picture-postcard vision of bilingualism with the meanness and pettiness that arose in response to Levine's appointment.

The 1960s saw an expansion in the Ottawa public service, followed by a policy of official bilingualism and a series of changes in government institutions, writes Fraser. The Grey Nuns quietly withdrew from administering their hospital, the Ottawa General, which remained more or less bilingual through its expansion. The Civic Hospital, by contrast, was thoroughly anglophone. The policy of bilingualism is now seen very differently in Ottawa depending on one's social class and professional level. Those at the executive level are provided with French training, unlike workers at the lower echelons who see bilingualism as a threat and an added barrier to employment and advancement. Despite Levine's assurances that not everyone will have to be bilingual, Fraser says that many remain convinced that his nomination sent the message that unilingual anglophones will be replaced by bilingual people, i.e., francophones.

They believe their workplace will be "Bilingual Today, French Tomorrow," to cite an anti-francophone tract of twenty-five years ago.

> I know it's unjust. Yes, there are anti-francophone groups and indi-
> viduals, and irresponsible journalists who feed and give life to these
> fears. But they exist, and they are deep. Don't forget that there is a
> considerable number of Ottawa residents who are former Montrealers
> who, like the Cubans of Miami, retain a ferocious nostalgia for a van-
> ished past.

These fears are an ongoing matter aside from Levine's political engagement of 1979 and are more widespread than one turbulent mob. Nevertheless, this fright-ful meeting and open display of hatred has had a positive effect; a great number of citizens opposed to Levine's nomination, when witness to this distressing sight, were shamed into backing off immediately. As Fraser sees it, there is a cosmopolitan community in Ottawa that is not interested in the parochial squab-bles; bureaucrats and university communities who are nervous in the face of such witch-hunts and sympathetic towards Levine. Fraser wishes Levine well in dealing with the combined problems of a bitterly divided community and a deficit of 36 million dollars.

Ottawa Citizen. The *Ottawa Citizen's* Outaouais columnist, Bob Phillips, apolo-gizes for writing yet another column on the Levine affair but feels that the problem of Quebec's insufficient payment for Ontario health services needs a closer look ("Quebec's unpaid health tab"—City editorial page). He first dis-sociates himself from those who use words like "traitor," saying that "some of the wild-eyed views committed to paper are embarrassing to anyone with a feeling for Canadian values." He also blames the federal government for turn-ing a "blind eye to this Quebec larceny, though the federal minister went bal-listic when Alberta threatened to deviate from the Canada Health Act by sup-porting private medicine." He thinks the Ontario hospitals should press their case against Quebec before the federal government. Phillips reiterates argu-ments made earlier by Dr. Charles Shaver, whom he acknowledges.

Concerning the medical services payments, Phillips suggests that Levine's past political connections with the governing Quebec party may produce a conflict of interest: "This is a proper question for a competent board. It implies no thought control or political censorship, and has little to do with national unity." Phillips also notes that, if Quebec separated, the cost for one day's stay in an Ontario hospital would be $2,000 to $3,000. In other words, if Levine were to live in a separate Quebec and yet be admitted to an Ontario hospital he would have to pay a four-fold increase. Hence, Phillips advises Levine to con-sider aiding confederation instead of separation.

An editorial-page article by Bill Shannon, an Ottawa writer, analyses the frustration that found a target in Levine ("Anglophone anger must be addressed"). Shannon sees the outburst as a valuable signal to Quebec that a breakup of Canada would not be amicable: "Don't be fooled that all will be sweetness and light if you separate, as your leaders tell you."

People are angry at the board membership, Shannon suggests, because they are the kind of people responsible for job loss through "right sizing." They are angry because the Montfort Hospital, a French language hospital, has been spared from closure. They see supposedly bilingual hospitals, such as the General and Elisabeth Bruyère, as francophone hospitals that tolerate anglophones. Many among the middle-aged crowd, brought up only in English, are angry because they were forced to take language training. In light of these points, the selection of a man who worked for a separatist government becomes understandable. "Tolerance" is a red herring, writes Phillips, a "cover up for the real causes of anger ... [that] have to be recognized and considered."

Le Journal de Montréal. Michel Auger, writing in *Le Journal de Montréal*, draws attention to divisions in the anglophone community. Alliance Quebec had issued a bulletin saying that Levine's political past should not prevent him from heading the Ottawa Hospital, but Alliance-Outaouais condemned the nomination.

Friday, May 29

Ottawa Sun. The *Ottawa Sun* devotes a whole page to Earl McRae's report of a nine-page open letter sent to Chair Nick Mulder of the Ottawa Hospital Board by MPP Garry Guzzo. A grim-faced Guzzo is shown holding up the first page of the letter, and a smaller photo of Mulder is inset at the bottom left. The letter is a series of questions and concerns. McRae says that the letter implies that the Ontario Progressive Conservative government may be unwilling to provide $440 million funding for the hospital this year.

Among other things, Guzzo's letter deals with the board's questionable competency, first in hiring Levine, and second in conducting the May 19 meeting in a room seating only 265 people. It also states that, although David Levine was supposed to "clear the air" at the May 15 press conference by declaring that he was no longer a separatist, he failed to do so. He had been involved in 1995 in the drafting of the sovereignist Declaration of Independence prior to the referendum and was evasive when asked whether he had taken an Oath of Allegiance to the Independent State of Quebec on taking up his New York job.

McRae mentions two stories about Levine that were later treated as false rumours by the hospital board:

> I've also been informed by a highly reliable source that at a recent hockey game in New York between the Rangers and a Canadian team, Levine stood for the American anthem, but sat for *O Canada*. Guzzo

won't confirm or deny the report, allegedly from a Manhattan lawyer, but Guzzo in his letter mentions "the fact that Mr. Levine has severe difficulty in standing for the Canadian national anthem when it is played."

This story was denied by the hospital board in its June 9 statement. Surely Guzzo, if his source is so knowledgeable and reliable, can give the date and time of the hockey game in question?

McRae continues:

> Guzzo says some of Levine's former hospital co-workers recall him speaking disparagingly about Canada, allegedly referring to Canada as a "disgrace and a joke," and Guzzo hits Mulder with this: "I don't expect you or any of your board to feel this strongly about people calling our country 'a joke' and a 'disgrace,' but, sir, maybe after the honor of the Order of Canada has rested on your shoulders a few more years, you, too, will find this distasteful."

This story, originally linked to the Montfort Hospital, was later challenged on the basis that Levine never worked at the Montfort. Continued circulation of this kind of story without providing evidence smacks of irresponsible journalism.

Le Devoir. A letter dated May 20 from Raynald Adams in *Le Devoir* defends Levine on the grounds that, until the "new order" (presumably a separate Quebec) is founded, Quebecers remain Canadians, paying taxes like other Canadians and being protected by the same Charter of Rights and Freedoms. Levine in 1979 and Raynald Adams today writing in favour of separatism are exercising rights accorded under Canadian law. "I don't believe," writes Adams, "that the violation of fundamental rights of David Levine are 'the price to pay for his political beliefs.'"

Le Droit. Gervais Pomerleau of Havre-Aubert submits a strongly worded letter to *Le Droit,* denouncing the "hypocrisy" in the "dirty Levine affair" and the "filthy" display of xenophobia targeted at half the population of Quebec. Why should Levine's ability to do the job be influenced by his past political beliefs? asks Pomerleau. Are they looking for someone to head a hospital or a Canadian unity centre? Compared to what has taken place regarding Levine, the "great Love-in" of October 1995 looks in retrospect like a fine bit of Canadian hypocrisy. Come the next referendum, Pomerleau will take into account the Quebec motto "Je me souviens!" (I remember).

Saturday May 30

Ottawa Sun. Once again Saturday's *Sun* devotes a lot of space to the Levine affair. David Frum suggests in his column, "Strange place to draw a line," that in the hardening of attitudes against and the repression of separatism in Canada, David Levine is an illogical focus for such activity. Many separatists are employed by the federal government, including employees of Radio Canada in particular. Lucien Bouchard once held a job as an ambassador and cabinet minister. Through transfer payments, Canada supports the Quebec education system, which promotes separatism. "If separatism really is sedition," writes Frum, "why are we fretting over the sympathies of hospital chiefs instead of purging the army, the RCMP, the Bank of Canada and other key agencies of persons of questionable loyalty?" If we are to move towards repression, there are mightier powers, such as the War Measures Act, to use. But we decided long ago that it made "more sense to win the referendum than to ban it, more sense to outtalk the separatists than to outfight them, more sense to bribe them than to punish them." If we maintain the path of conciliation, "then David Levine should be permitted to do his job in peace." Frum denies, however, that political beliefs are irrelevant to employment, claiming that politically correct views on feminism, gay rights, multiculturalism and a "host of other favored causes" is "virtually a precondition for any important taxpayer-funded job in this country." Frum's column also appears the same day in the *Financial Post.*[2]

Once again Earl McRae acts as cheerleader for the anti-Levine forces, reporting that MPP Garry Guzzo received more than three hundred phone calls of support after the *Sun* published his open letter to Nick Mulder. McRae scorned Mulder's reported remark to Guzzo May 6 that the anti-separatist controversy would just "blow over in a weekend." He also encourages those opposed to the board and Levine to attend the board's next meeting on June 6. The Alliance for the Preservation of English in Canada (APEC) is mentioned as an organizing body, with telephone numbers given for George Potter and Tony Silvestro. Wade Wallace, an ex-Quebecer, also invited phone calls from parties interested in forming an organization for developing strategies to combat the Levine appointment. "It's your serve," concluded McRae.

A letter from Arnold Kaleta protested former Ottawa Mayor Marion Dewar's support for the board when a majority of people at the May 19 public meeting were opposed to the board's decision.

Monday, May 31

Ottawa Sun. Two letters appeared in the Sunday *Sun.* Andre Perras of Kanata protests against paying a "king's ransom" to "a man who would usurp another's freedoms." He suggests, in language contrasting Levine with Perras's ancestor (who left his home country for Canada), that Levine has behaved in a cowardly way by not leaving the country he has sought to split up. Perras also criticizes Earl McRae, however, for describing the Montfort fight to survive as "petulant": "Congratulations, Earl. You are the separatists' means to their odious end."

Joe Houlden addresses his note to rights defenders, saying that, in the absence of a law affirming the indivisibility of Canada, they owe a debt to the rednecks for ensuring that "David Levine and other separatists do not operate with the total impunity that you are illogically willing to grant them."

Le Devoir. *Le Devoir* keeps attention on the Levine affair with an analysis of the English-language press and a review of an article written by Ernest Cadegan for the Halifax *Daily News.* Cadegan says that the outburst in Ottawa was occasioned by the longterm impact of official bilingualism, which Ottawans feel is a painful plague. This tension caused by bilingualism was accentuated by budgetary cuts, "the unending national unity crisis and the inflammatory and dishonest rhetoric of the Quebec sovereignty movement." This doesn't justify but explains the reaction of people in Ottawa and should make us aware of one thing: "The Canada-Quebec divorce can only be a rancorous event."

Cadegan also argues that tolerance becomes a form of decadence when it is not founded on any solid belief. Tolerance in this case may just be opting out. Those who protest the nomination of a separatist are showing their intolerance for someone who would break up the country, and that's not necessarily a bad thing, he says.

• • •

June and July

Significant developments in the David Levine affair continue to take place after the intense period in the latter part of May. The election of William "Pit Bill" Johnson to the leadership of Alliance Quebec, which most aggressively defends English rights in Quebec, has led to reflections on Franco-Canadian rights elsewhere in Ontario. The Levine case is often mentioned by the French language media as an example of anglo intolerance outside Quebec.

Ottawa Sun. The June 2 *Ottawa Sun* devotes over half a page to a protest on June 1, including a picture of 80-year-old Kay Clancy carrying a "Separatists, Traitors" placard. The story by Sarah Green notes that the angry mood of the meeting was reminiscent of the May 19 meeting, except that this time questions from the public were answered by chair Nick Mulder. Dozens of people were excluded from the small room, though, and protester Ray Grant stormed in during a presentation about local cancer services and began shouting and angrily pounding the table. As police escorted him out he shouted "Love your country. What does it take to love your country," Green reports.

Earl McRae continues his cheerleading with a column on June 8, "Keep on fighting hospital board." He begins:

> Voiceless, helpless, frustrated, powerless. That's how you good and caring citizens are feeling in your efforts to go up against the intransigent Ottawa Hospital board and its political power backers in the fiasco appointment of the separatist David Levine to CEO of the newly amalgamated hospital.

McRae urges his followers to "keep chipping away at the ankles of the insolent giant that believes it can't be toppled." He counsels them not to stop faxing board members, cancelling hospital donations however small, and boycotting businesses of board members. He proposes that the goal no longer be to unseat Levine, but to pressure the Ontario government for a provincial law to ensure that the board will be elected the same as school boards.

Le Droit. On June 2, *Le Droit* also devotes nearly three-quarters of a page to the meeting on the previous day. "Less numerous, but always as virulent," reads the headline. Isabelle Ducas estimates the crowd at 250 and notes that Ron Leitch, president of the Alliance for the Preservation of English in Canada (APEC) came up from Toronto to address the board. About fifty members of APEC attended, she writes. She describes the two protesters who were escorted out by police. One black man denied that he was a redneck: "My neck is black, but I love my country. What does it take for you to love your country?" he reportedly asked. The other person interrupted the budget presentation to say "And the separatist. How much will he cost?" Several people objected to the use of French among the board members. "In English, please! It's an English meeting and it's an English region," several people reportedly said. A woman continued, "These bastards! Speak English, and if you don't like it go back to Quebec. That's what will happen if we do nothing, they will dictate to us."

Ottawa Citizen. Several organizations continued to press for the removal of Levine. Demonstrations at the regular meetings of the Ottawa Hospital board of trustees continued, with consequent news coverage. The June 16 *Ottawa Citizen* carried three columns of copy, five inches deep, in its City section along with a 7 inch by 4 inch picture of an angry woman. This meeting was particularly significant—the first one in which David Levine appeared as the new CEO.

Dave Ebner's story, "Angry crowd greets Levine," emphasizes the storm of insults, including one directed at a *Citizen* photographer who was called a "separatist b-tch" as she snapped pictures of the event. The picture that made its way into the paper could hardly be said to reflect favourably on the demonstrators. Anger was generated partly from the fact that only thirty-four members of the public were allowed into the boardroom at the Civic site's Parkdale clinic, while about seventy-five were left outside struggling against police and security. Nicholas Patterson, a regular protester at many meetings, was also outside organizing boycotts of board members' businesses, Ebner reported.

Le Devoir. An interesting letter by Augustin Roy appears in *Le Devoir* on June 3, calling into question the right of the Parti Québécois government to condemn the "intolerance" shown to Levine. Just as the people of Ottawa want a CEO who shares their vision of Canada, so does the PQ government in relation to its ideology, writes Roy.

He cites the appointment of Rosette Côté to the position of commissioner for complaints regarding health and social services as a particularly glaring example of patronage. "It's easier to condemn others than to honestly assess one's own conduct. Intolerance on the one side begets fanaticism in the others," he concludes.

JUNE 15 PROTEST

Ottawa Sun. The June 16 *Sun* carries a front-page headline in one-inch bold type: "Raucous start for Levine." The story by Sarah Green reports that cries of "Shame!" greeted David Levine as he took his seat with the board after his first day on the job. The reporter judges the number of people excluded from the meeting to be more than one hundred. Inside the paper a full page is devoted to the story, and a picture shows police officers in a relaxed mood while placards reading "Democracy abused—Dictators" and "Levine resign" are displayed by protesters. A small photo of a somewhat displeased-looking David Levine is shown. In an inset story, Green describes events at the General site of the new Ottawa Hospital, focusing on a new birth as a symbol of business as usual, regardless of the new appointment ("Levine's first day fails to make an impression").

Le Droit. *Le Droit* also gives a lengthy report on the June 15 protest, identifying George Potter as an organizer of a "Save the Civic" meeting and a member of APEC. Reporter Isabelle Ducas also names Bill Halliday as a speaker who told Levine that people would be better served by his leaving: "Go somewhere else to do your work of breaking up the country. You are not welcome here," he reportedly said.

Ottawa Sun. The *Sun* carries a story on the Ottawa Hospital board's complaint that the protests are slowing down important work that needs to be done ("Board sick of protest," June 17, p. 10). On the same day, an editorial, calling for more civility in the protesting, argues that "National unity is not advanced one bit when francophones are branded as traitorous separatists. And that's what happened during Monday's noisy confrontation." The antics were by a very few people but "their small numbers are having an enormous impact nonetheless in distorting the real and more credible opposition to Levine's appointment."

Picketing of Businesses. Apart from protest meetings, the other main development is the picketing of businesses associated with board members. One target is Barbara Ramsay, owner of a local Shoppers Drug Mart.

Ottawa Citizen. Nathan Vardi's news story of June 21, "Ramsay targeted for fourth day," reports that about thirty people marched outside Barbara Ramsay's Shopper Drug Mart at Merivale Mall on Saturday. Ramsay is reported as saying, "I empathize with these people, but I am not going to resign. It is very difficult to make the correlation and explain this to my employees and I am concerned with my livelihood and the livelihood of 45 employees."

Two groups were involved in the picketing: Unity Canada and a "grass roots movement without a name," Vardi writes. David Green, an organizer with Unity Canada, stated that his group had a protest permit and were "not making a personal attack on Barbara Ramsay." Speaking for the other group was the ubiquitous Nicholas Patterson. Patterson reportedly said his movement was assembling about seven thousand leaflets that urge people to leave Bell Telephone for a competitor because of Nick Mulder's connection to that company.

Opinion supporting David Levine and the hospital board gets a powerful boost in the *Ottawa Citizen* on June 25. A front-page story in the City section by Maria Bohuslawsky ("Former mayors praise Levine"), focuses on a meeting between two former mayors of Ottawa, Jacquelin Holzman and Jim Durrell, and David Levine, at the end of which both Holzman and Durrell were full of praise and confidence in the new CEO. Since both figures have their roots in the anglophone community of Ottawa, their views will likely carry a lot of weight with the public.

Three letters against the boycott and in defence of Barbara Ramsay are also printed the same day under the heading "Boycotting store of hospital trustee makes no sense." The letters, by Lisa Miller, Lisa Stromquist and Benita Siemiatycki, are very articulate and takes up thirty-two column inches. Lisa Miller writes as an employee at Barbara Ramsay's Shoppers Drug Mart to complain about people coming into the store yelling "You people are working for a separatist." Performing the duties of a pharmacy technician can be quite hectic, and "the last thing I need is to have to fend off people who are angry with Barbara, especially when the issue has no bearing on my job," she says. "*Barbara Ramsay is not a separatist.* Maybe some of you should back up and read that sentence again."

Lisa Stromquist, another employee of the targeted Shoppers Drug Mart, complains that her ability to serve the public as a health care professional has been "hindered by the barrage of telephone calls, faxes and interruptions by irate individuals who don't seem to understand that targeting this store will do nothing to change the appointment of David Levine." The protesters are "distorting facts" in "calling Barbara Ramsay a separatist," creating a great deal of confusion. Stromquist asks the protesters to "remember to look at the faces of those you are hurting on our way to work."

Benita Siemiatycki is seeking the names and places of work or business ownership of the individuals calling for the boycott of Barbara Ramsay's Shoppers Drug Mart. In that way those who are "sickened by the intimidation and bigotry demonstrated by those opposed to David Levine's appointment" can respond in kind. She mentions that Ramsay risked her own safety during the ice storm to deliver prescriptions to rural residents trapped in their homes. "From what I observe," writes Siemiatycki, the individuals involved in the protest

> are a loud and obnoxious minority who are using harassment and intimidation to get the attention of the board when it has a hugely important decision to make about the health care of this community. Their propaganda is extremely divisive, and may take years from which to recover.

As a former Montrealer, Siemiatycki says she is able to

> know the difference between a hard-core separatist and an anglophone who simply respects French Quebecers' desire to have autonomy if they so choose democratically, and doesn't see it as the end of the world. It is time the *Citizen* stopped giving exposure to the narrow-minded and destructive views of a vocal minority, especially when it impacts so negatively on the community.

The *Citizen* reports a continuation of the boycott June 29, with the announcement that a protest group called Operation Boycott/Picket, organized by Nicholas Patterson, will picket the office of real estate broker and Ottawa Hospital trustee Sol Shinder that same day. Patterson told the newspaper his group wants to picket all twelve private business of the board of trustees of the Ottawa Hospital.

Ottawa Sun. More coverage of the boycott is provided in the *Ottawa Sun* on June 21, with a large picture of a protester standing next to a Canadian flag outside the Merivale Shoppers Drug Mart. Cliff Parmeter, Tony Silvestro, Carol Dane, Nicholas Patterson and David Green are named among the group of about twenty protesters. Kathleen Harris's story reports Barbara Ramsay as being supportive of peaceful protest but says she is "tremendously saddened by the violence" that has erupted in the last few days. "The methodology used is overwhelmingly negative and not helpful," Ramsay says.

APEC. The Alliance for the Preservation of English in Canada takes out an advertisement in the *Sun* on June 18. Measuring 7 inches by 12 inches, it says "If 'improving health care' means disrupting the community and losing millions in donations, Premier Harris is doing a great job." The advertisement includes a coupon soliciting donations to APEC and asking respondents to indicate whether they did or did not "support an English-speaking hospital for Ottawa—the nation's capital, and whether they did or did not agree that "The Hospital Board must resign." A second advertisement appears in the *Ottawa Citizen* on June 23. This time it reads "Premier Harris, in Ottawa you are playing politics with hospitals and people's lives. Why?" It is accompanied by the same coupon.

The president of APEC, Ronald Leitch, writes to the *Financial Post* on June 4 to rebut a *Post* editorial from May 26 upholding David Levine's human rights. "No one is denying Levine the right to work. What is being denied is his right to hold a government job at taxpayers' expense in Ontario."

Those looking for an end to the turmoil were relieved at the conciliatory attitude shown in the *Sun's* July 3 editorial ("Heal"). David Levine is noted as having chosen Chris Carruthers, a unilingual anglophone, as his chief of staff. "By choosing Carruthers, Levine and the board signal two things: One, that the Civic retains a key role in this new hospital. Two, that bilingualism is not a chief of staff's prime qualification," editorializes the *Sun*. The newspaper is happy that the community concerns are finally being addressed: "Better late than never. To us, it just shows the power ordinary citizens can wield when they have the courage to speak out."

Le Droit. Just as the *Sun* is coming to approve of Levine's actions, *Le Droit* begins to wonder whether Levine's hands will be tied by the ever-present crowd of people hostile to any increase in French in the region's institutions. The question among the French-speaking population is whether their right to treatment in their own language will be respected, now that the Montfort Hospital's services are to be reduced.

Notes

1. Contrary to Fotheringham's claim, newspapers in other parts of Canada were supportive of keeping Levine, as excerpts in this chapter prove.
2. One answer to David Frum's article was provided on June 3 in a letter to the *Sun* by MPP Garry Guzzo, who writes that the reason there was a fuss made in this case, as distinct from the senior federal positions occupied by separatists, is that Levine's salary was paid for by Ontario tax dollars.

CHAPTER FIVE

OVERVIEW, ANALYSIS AND EVALUATION

So many issues coalesced around the David Levine affair that it is a challenge simply to sort out the different factors at play. Though Canadians are faced with problems and choices—health care, provincial and federal deficits, the national debt, bilingualism, support for multiculturalism—in the Ottawa area, Canadian unity is a prominent concern. It is tied more closely to people's jobs, their lives and the value of their homes than elsewhere in the country. Memories of the razor-edged federalist victory in the 1995 referendum contribute to strong emotional reactions against separatism and indifference to the separatist threat. For many who feel that the federal government did not do enough to promote national unity, the appointment of David Levine was a spark that lit the fire of grassroots protest. At his appearance, groups anxious to make their views known and heeded become organized, and those already in existence, such as the implausibly named Alliance for the Preservation of English in Canada, grew in prominence.

Antipathy to separatism was, on the face of things, the most important nerve touched by the Levine appointment. But there were others. In Ontario, the Progressive Conservative government of Mike Harris pushed restructuring of the local hospital system, despite strong campaigns to save existing hospitals. Resentment for what is widely perceived as bureaucratic insensitivity has been building in the community, while the Health Services Restructuring Commission juggernaut crashed through the impasse to announce its final directives on August 13, 1997—the merger of the Civic, General and Riverside Hospitals, and the transfer of some programs from the Grace and Montfort Hospitals. This was followed by a Transition Steering Committee, formed in late 1997 to develop criteria for the new CEO of the amalgamated Ottawa Hospital, and the Ottawa Hospital Board of Trustees, formed on April 1, 1998.

The restructuring was designed to bring efficiencies and economies to the health care system. Modern techniques in medicine have reduced the length of hospital stays, and persuasive arguments have indicated that costs could be further reduced by closing some hospitals to fill up beds in others. Also, by consolidating high-tech equipment used in treatment or research in one institution, duplication can be avoided. But the desire for "efficiency" has also meant that health care has become less rewarding. Staff are overworked and frequently rotated, to the detriment of patient care.[1] Emergency wards are overcrowded.

Alongside technical questions are sociopolitical concerns. How does one ensure that unilingual patients get treated in their own language when they are required to attend a hospital in which the staff speaks the other language, or predominantly so? How does one ensure, in a bilingual hospital, that patients feel comfortable with staff members who are not bilingual or who converse among themselves in the other official language? Elderly patients in particular, who often feel helpless as their lives are entrusted to the system, may encounter the additional strangeness of an unfamiliar language and hence great insecurity.

The Franco-Ontarian community felt this way when closure of the Montfort Hospital was threatened. After a huge rally at the Civic Centre in Ottawa assurances were given that the Hospital would stay open. Some among the anglophone community resented what they saw as another special favour to the French. Meanwhile, the French-speaking population has been wondering whether services at the Montfort will be so reduced in scope that it won't be recognizable as the same hospital.

In a June 1998 interview Ottawa Hospital Board Chair Nick Mulder listed the six main concerns behind the opposition to the board: (1) separatism; (2) the respective roles of the Civic (previously English-speaking) and General (bilingual) hospital sites; (3) bilingualism; (4) the role of the French-speaking Montfort Hospital; (5) hospital jobs, especially for unilingual staff; and (6) fee differentials between Ontario and Quebec, and collecting full Ontario fees for treatment of Quebec residents.[2] The following expands on these and other issues.

Separatism. Most people in Ottawa are strongly federalist. When the Parti Québécois nearly won the October 1995 referendum, what had been a mere theory became a tangible threat to livelihood and identity. Many realized what might be lost with a separate Quebec and wondered whether it was a good idea to simply do nothing and say nothing, leaving everything to Quebec, when their own well-being was at stake. These feelings lacked an appropriate outlet.

Rumour that a loyal péquiste was going to be working from within Ontario, as head of the Ottawa Hospital, to promote separatism understandably produced an uproar. It was bad enough that federal taxes support the separatist party and its many followers in the civil service, but this position is paid from Ontario taxpayers' money.

The idea that Levine is bent on promoting separatism in Ontario is ill-founded and highly prejudicial. Looking at his background as a whole, the pattern of activity supports his claim that his main career goal is hospital administration. When, Levine declined on principle to reveal his beliefs about separatism, other than that he believed in the right of Quebecers to determine their future democratically, this prejudice was reinforced. Knowing from the start that Levine's CEO job would not allow him to put politics ahead of the best interests of the hospital and the community might have reduced some of the public tensions, but it would have been a mistake to think that this was the protesters' only concern. For some, it was enough that Levine had run for the PQ in 1979. He became, for these people, a symbol of what had caused much angst in their lives. Others who did not share this kind of concern, nonetheless recognized these strong feelings as lack of support and confidence for Levine in the community, and they objected to the appointment for that reason.

There were other divisions in opinion. For some people, a 19-year-old commitment to the PQ, later rejected, might have been forgiven. But Levine had recently been appointed delegate general to New York—hardly a non-political appointment, since the previous delegate had been a Liberal who resigned after his party lost power. For many, this proved his belief in the separatist cause. In their view, he had done something appalling—setting out to break up Canada. They felt that he owed it to the community to at least disavow his presumed attachment to separatism, not be rewarded with a plum job paying $330,000 a year of Ontario taxpayers' money.

At the meetings, some individuals showed an anti-French bias, complaining, for example, when French was spoken. But others took pains to deny that they were anti-French—anti-separatist but not anti-French, they said. George Potter, an organizer and letter writer objected to separatist intolerance of the English in Quebec and said that he could not support anyone who was in league with a party that denies fundamental rights. He is married to a French-Canadian, has a French-speaking daughter and has no anti-French feeling but, as further questioning revealed, he is not happy with imposed bilingualism and did not seem put out by my suggestion that a strong opposition to Levine might encourage separation. He described that outcome as preferable to a two-faced position of gains and power for the French in the rest of Canada and autonomy in Quebec. Many of the people I interviewed strongly resented the high proportion of francophones in the federal government, which gives Quebec more power than its numbers would warrant relative to the rest of Canada. This has often been treated as a necessary price to pay for Canadian unity, but the feeling among people like George Potter is that the price has become too high, particularly when so many Quebec francophones have simultaneously been seeking sovereignty.

The polling company COMPAS carried out a survey commissioned by the *Ottawa Citizen*, which was published on May 18. The survey showed that Ottawa residents were evenly divided over the question whether David Levine should be "forced to resign"—56 percent lacked confidence in the committee that selected Levine. The question drew attention to both Levine's separatism and his previous experience as a hospital administrator, but it did not bring into play how Quebec opinion might react to a decision to rescind the Levine appointment. The May 15–16 survey was useful and important, but it caught opinion at a time when the media was most strongly focused on Levine's past separatist connections rather than on his break with the PQ a few years after his candidacy. The survey correctly drew attention to the depth of feeling among anti-Levine people, which was greater than that of the pro-Levine camp. But opinion was skewed by the anti-Levine media and by the way in which Levine's unwillingness to divulge his private political beliefs, which may have been a principled freedom-of-belief stand, was interpreted.

Iona Skuce, a retired economist and public servant, on hearing of my study on the Levine controversy, informed me that she had conducted about two hundred interviews with the public, including physicians and dentists. Since her study was done in the course of her daily activities, it could hardly be described as scientific because the results could reflect opinion only in her particular milieu. About 90 percent of interviewees were against the appointment, she found. A senior physician argued that anyone who would choose separatism showed bad judgement, and therefore Levine ought not to have been selected. Interviewees frequently objected to having "their tax dollars going to the cause of the separatists," she said, adding that the words "bilingual" and "French" were never mentioned.[3] The reference to the separatist "cause," suggests that these respondents were under the impression that Levine would continue to promote separatism while holding the Ottawa job. That assumption ought to have been laid to rest early in the affair. But the way in which some of the local media presented Levine lent this assumption inordinate tenacity in the first few weeks of May.

People would be right to object to the head of an Ontario hospital putting the politics of separatism above the best interests of the medical job to which he or she is appointed. Political impartiality has been recognized as a necessary feature of public employment. The Employee Code of Conduct for the Regional Municipality of Ottawa-Carleton states "To ensure public trust in the RMOC, employees must be, and appear to be, both politically impartial and free of undue political influence in the exercise of their duties."[4] Levine made it quite clear, early on, that his political beliefs would not affect his job. The question, however, should have focused on whether this assurance was sufficient; in the light of rumours and prejudicial information, it did not seem so. The community was asked to trust Levine, trust the hospital board and trust Chair Nick Mulder. Against a background of mistrust engendered by the Harris government's fondness for government by decree rather than respect for due process and participatory democracy, this was a tall order.[5]

For some, trust was not the issue. The extremists against the "softness" on the "Quebec question" have treated separatism as if it were treason and separatists as if they were tainted by criminality, regardless of what the law might provide. Such a view conflicts with existing Canadian opinion, though. Why else would we accept the existence of the Bloc Québécois and the Parti Québécois? Because Canadians seek solutions to political problems in a democratic way. As long as these parties are legitimate, people who adhere to their policies and objectives will be protected under the freedoms cited in Sections

2(b) and 2(d) of the Canadian Charter of Rights and Freedoms. Such tolerant attitudes are a target for extremists, and how Canadians respond to their challenge will affect the character of this country.

Without necessarily adopting the extremist standpoint, some Canadians argue that there has been too much accommodation of the abstract arguments of separatists and not enough thinking about the adverse consequences of a possible separation on people's lives and on the economy. Many feel that the dream of an easy separation, however attractive, is unrealistic in the light of resultant economic disadvantages. Others use the language of "appeasement," evoking Chamberlain's attempt to pacify Hitler prior to the Second World War and referring obliquely to Quebec's language laws and threats of violence towards those who are not acquiescent to separatist aspirations.

A less tendentious word for "appeasement" would be "accommodation." Judging by the many concessions granted to Quebec over the past decades, it would appear that Canadians have been willing, with differing levels of enthusiasm perhaps, to support Quebec's aspirations to preserve and promote its French language and culture. The experience of the October Crisis of 1970 solidified Canadians' preference for democratic ways in which Quebecers may choose their destiny. But that does not dispel the feeling in English Canada that it has given too many concessions to Quebec and that Quebec has not reciprocated sufficiently, having retained its restrictive language laws. Since the federal government's 1970 adoption of official bilingualism, the francophone presence has grown considerably in the civil service. Massive federal buildings were constructed on the Quebec side of the Ottawa River to improve the Quebec economy and establish a federal presence there. These concessions were made to improve the likelihood of Quebecers wanting to remain within confederation. A substantial number of the Quebec population, however, wants nothing short of full sovereignty. No concessions will ever be sufficient, and each new concession merely shortens the distance to the goal. For federalists in the rest of Canada, it is an exercise in frustration, the likes of which is exploited on radio phone-in programs by hosts who ask listeners what kind of wimps and suckers they are to stand for an arrangement that amounts to blackmail. The quasi-separatist position of "Give us more or we'll leave" is not the kind of attitude that engenders sympathy.

Given this history, the appointment of David Levine appears as yet another concession, a way of saying, "You can try to break up Canada, but you are still entitled to the rights of any Canadian, so come and take a plum Ontario job." Many (and not just the boisterous crowd) believe that loyalty matters. And if you are disloyal to a system, it seems wrong to benefit from that system.

One answer to this last point is that it is never disloyal to seek to improve a system in ways that are countenanced by that system. In some cases, such as civil disobedience, a citizen may feel that loyalty requires going beyond what is officially countenanced by the system. Interestingly, it was an agitator against

David Levine and the hospital board, Earl McRae, who supported civil disobedience. The big divide occurs between those who think that a sovereign Quebec would be an improvement over the existing political system and those who don't. The arguments for and against have resonated in discussions about Levine.

Some believe that Quebec separation would introduce more—and more serious—problems than those we now face. What about English-speaking enclaves of people who prefer to keep their Canadian passports? What about the territorial claims of aboriginal peoples in Quebec? All kinds of existing arrangements would need to be re-negotiated with the rest of Canada. Opponents say that none of these problems is insuperable, and that only when sovereignty is achieved can the French Quebecer feel like a first-class citizen instead of a member of the minority. Somewhere between these two extremes are the many Canadians who don't feel that just because one group is in the majority, the minority must be made to feel like second-class citizens. Enacting safeguards to protect minority rights can make them feel like a recognized part of the larger society.

That is the challenge of Canada, a goal that was promoted by Pierre Elliot Trudeau as Prime Minister and one that has in some respects succeeded admirably to this point. It brought with it a policy of increased bilingualism, which many welcomed at first, enrolling their English-speaking children in French immersion classes. There were also disillusionments. And cases of unfair advancement of some individuals over others, giving undue weight to the bilingual factor, became legendary.

Bilingualism. Levine was perceived by many as likely to promote bilingualism in the Ottawa Hospital in the same way that bilingualism had been promoted in the federal government. Those unilingual anglophones whose careers had been blocked in the federal government or those who had left Montreal because of their language handicap, would see the same disadvantages, instituted in Ottawa and paid for by Ontario dollars, as most unpalatable.

As mentioned earlier, not everyone took into account that the policy of bilingualism in the Ottawa Hospital was set by the Ottawa Hospital board and that Levine's job was solely to implement it. Nevertheless, perhaps it was assumed that he would follow the policy enthusiastically. In this case the wishes of a number of anglophones conflict with those of the francophone population; the former wish Levine would drag his feet and the latter naturally want to see French patients served for all ailments, at whichever hospital site treatment might be needed, in their own language.

In speaking with protesters against the Levine appointment, it became clear to me that a substantial number of them seemed to want a unilingual English-speaking Ontario. When it was pointed out to them that their desire is the same as that of Quebecers who seek a unilingual French-speaking Quebec, and that this would give further support to separatism, some accepted this outcome with equanimity. They were quite prepared to accept a separate Quebec as a preferable alternative to bilingualism elsewhere in Canada. Why then condemn separatism? Why the slogans "Down with separatism" and "Separatists go home"?

The answer seems partly that the individuals in question don't like the ambiguity of the present situation, wherein the face of Quebec is both federalist and separatist. They believe that, in the name of federalism and accommodation, English Canada makes concessions inside and outside of Quebec. But wherever the Quebec government exercises its power, it tends to promote separatism, in education in particular—hence the hatred for the PQ policies, which extends to those who have supported them and perhaps still do. Placing this situation in a historical context might help extremists to temper their hatred and to understand that in Quebec, prior to the Quiet Revolution, unilingual francophones were at a disadvantage in competing for top jobs in an English-dominated society and economy. Those who feel insulted because the apostrophe has been dropped from Eaton's might consider how typical it was in the earlier days for English media to drop the accents from French words. Attempts to redress the balance need to be understood, even when particular measures may overshoot the mark.

To the above-mentioned visceral antipathies to separatism I add the fear that David Levine is an ardent, dyed-in-the-wool separatist who will do everything to cause disruption and confusion. The most extreme conspiracy theorists perhaps feel that Lucien Bouchard had a clever scheme to get Levine in power, allow him to create enough disruption to be fired and thereby provide Bouchard with an excuse to say that the rest of Canada is intolerant of Quebecers. Perhaps this would swing "soft" federalists over to the sovereignty camp in enough numbers to win the next referendum. To the extent that the media portrayed David Levine as a PQ stalwart, originally on a top mission to New York and perhaps still in league with the party, they encouraged this kind of thinking early on. It remains one of the major misunderstandings about Levine.

Fee Differentials. Objection to the Levine appointment was also tied to Quebec's failure to respect fully the provisions of the Canada Health Act, which require that when patients from one province are treated in another, the province of residence should pay according to the fee schedule charged by the host province. Quebec, however, commonly pays other provinces only at rates charged in its own system. By special agreement in certain areas, Ottawa being one, Quebec will provide full payment, but for a limited range of cases and under limited circumstances. Dr. Charles Shaver of Nepean has for many years carried out a public education campaign to promote full portability of medical coverage throughout Canada. He has published letters and articles in Quebec and elsewhere calling attention to the isolation facing those of limited means should Quebec separate. He would like to see the federal government take action to enforce the Canada Health Act provisions. Similar concerns have led some to view the Levine appointment negatively, on the grounds that Levine will be likely to use his influence to further Quebec's interests. As has been mentioned, however, such a policy is handled by the Ontario and Quebec health ministries and is not part of the Ottawa Hospital CEO's responsibility.

Implications of Acquiescence. A sophisticated reckoning of the use to which Levine's appointment might be put by separatist propaganda is another cause for concern. David Kwavnick, a political scientist formerly of Carleton University, articulated the point to me in private correspondence. Part of the case Lucien Bouchard would like to present to Quebecers who are hesitating over the separatist option is that separation will be painless and that the rest of Canada is not really concerned. Wrote Kwavnick:

> If the Levine appointment is allowed to stand simply because he was the best qualified candidate for the job it will mean that the rest of us do not have strong feelings about separatism and that our only interest is, indeed, to ensure business as usual. In any future referendum it will be cited up and down Quebec as proof that the rest of the country will agree to continue existing economic arrangements and that there will be no economic price to pay for separatism. And it will be an effective argument. That's why Bouchard intervened—to help save an important separatist argument—not to help promote Canadian unity.

That Lucien Bouchard would not have intervened for the sake of Canadian unity seems a plausible supposition. And it may well be true that those who protested so vehemently against Levine's appointment may have accomplished something worthwhile for federalism, namely to organize a strong opposition to the breakup of Canada and to clarify that "business as usual" is not a foregone conclusion. But there is another side to Kwavnick's case. When Trudeau made his pitch for federalism in the 1960s, it was on the basis that Quebecers had much more to gain by being part of vast territory from coast to coast than by isolating themselves. For Trudeau's case to succeed francophones must feel welcome outside Quebec, without having to assimilate. Already the noisy protest of May 19 and remarks by Premier Mike Harris belied that sense of welcome. Termination of Levine's appointment, however, would have had a much more potent effect on opinion in Quebec. This is demonstrated in editorials and commentary in the French-language media and acknowledged by Ottawa-Carleton Regional Councillors Clive Doucet and Alex Munter and by Alliance Quebec leader William Johnson. Munter's view was poignantly stated in a letter addressed to the Ottawa Hospital board, May 21, 1998:

> Revoking Mr. Levine's appointment after some people say that members of a legal political party are "criminals" and should be arrested or

after others speak darkly of a francophone conspiracy to "take over," is wrong.

The issue has become symbolic and it has become national in significance. To fire Mr. Levine primarily because of his past political affiliations, after determining through a nation-wide search that you felt he was the best candidate for the job, would be difficult to justify. It would send the message to all Canadians that there is no hope for this country, that we cannot work together. It would be a particularly wrong statement for the nation's capital to make.

Erosion of Good Medical Care. Some resentment of the Levine appointment has little to do with the man himself and a lot to do with erosion of the health care system in Canada—steady cutbacks to health and education, and hospital restructuring generally. Insecurity about health, language and religion arises when hospitals with differing religious and linguistic backgrounds are placed under centralized control. One might have thought that having Jew as head of the hospital would at least provide a neutral party among the Catholics and Protestants. Likewise, having an anglophone who speaks French also makes it seem as though both linguistic groups would have their concerns met. The way Levine was presented by the media, however, depicted him as a turncoat against his own people in Montreal, someone who would serve the people in power without too much concern for the finer points of human rights. Hence some of the anglophone population feared that Levine would do the bidding of the vocal and active francophone minority in Ottawa-Carleton.

The insecurity felt in the region, especially among the elderly, should not be trivialized or underestimated. Regional Councillor Clive Doucet explained that his office regularly heard medical horror stories. For example, one elderly person was kept waiting at a hospital from 9 a.m. to 12 midnight with no one able to treat her swollen foot. Hospital staff tried to send her home, but she protested that she lived alone and could not walk. They sent her home the next day and provided two hours of home care when she really needed eighteen hours. She had to hire a private nurse.

Numerous stories about hospital incompetence and insensitivity have been making the rounds, unsurprising when many dedicated nurses have left public health care for private care or have left the profession entirely because of the inability to relate to patients on adequate human terms. By seeking maximum "efficiencies" in the system, the rewarding side of this profession has steadily diminished over the years. The assembly line is not geared to bringing out human qualities of compassion and understanding. The remaining staff is simply overworked and frustrated.

It is outside the scope of this book to delve into the politics behind the problems of restructuring, but a brief comment may be in order. There is a fairly widespread fear that the neo-conservative agenda involves abandoning

the national health care system in Canada in favour of a two-tier system ben-
efiting the rich; the model is Britain's Thatcherite system of siphoning the best
health care facilities for those able to pay. Private insurance companies would
protect the moderately wealthy from the sudden economic impact of an illness.
Those who think such a system would pose no problems might reflect on the
possibility of insurers picking and choosing among the candidates for insurance, so as not to be burdened with those in chronic need of expensive care.
This is the kind of thing that the Canadian system has avoided in the past. But
with the appearance of a more selfish, acquisitive society, it may be that the
influential segment of Canadian society no longer has the same commitment
and concern for the society as a whole. The trend to globalization has increased
the power of private enterprise to exert influence over government policies,
not surprisingly in the direction of profits and reduced taxes rather than egali-
tarian ideals. As Ottawa-Carleton Regional Councillor Clive Doucet put it:
"Withdrawing money from public service—that's what globalization is all
about."

So once again, it appears that the anxiety bursting to the surface in the
resentment against David Levine's appointment is only a symptom of much
more generalized insecurities. Levine symbolized for many in Ottawa a certain insensitivity to the feelings of the people, just one more manifestation of a
whole range of unconcerns. Through no fault of his own, David Levine became the target for this kind of underlying frustration and insecurity. People
seem to find that agitating against an individual is more feasible and emotion-
ally satisfying than targeting the more elusive forces that bear the real responsibility for their problems.

Scapegoat for Underlying Political Problems. David Levine is a useful scapegoat. It benefits Mike Harris that such a scapegoat exists. Outrage over his
appointment deflects attention away from the deficiencies of the whole restructuring process and the speedy timetable imposed by the Harris government. If things go wrong in the Ottawa Hospital, it can be blamed on the Levine
appointment, which in turn was made by the hospital board and not directly
under Harris's control. After all, Premier Harris distanced himself from responsibility, saying he would not have approved the hiring, but that he did not
have the power to overturn the appointment. Conservative MPP Garry Guzzo
was one of the prime movers seeking Levine's resignation and his comments
provided fuel for the highly emotional reaction. As early as May 8, he was
quoted in the *Citizen* as saying that Levine would fill "the whole administration with separatists" and that the "entire administration is going to have a
political agenda to break up the country." When I interviewed Guzzo on July
17 he said he did not believe what he was quoted as saying, though he did not
deny having said it. He told me that he had had evidence that Levine was going
to hire someone whom he knew from Quebec, someone who might or might

not have been a separatist. Guzzo's evidence was based mainly on the general tendency of people in power to hire those they know and trust. The person in question decided not to come in view of the furore that had been created, Guzzo said.

The Media

So far previous chapters have examined the day-by-day development of an explosive reaction to David Levine's appointment. This chapter has looked at underlying causes for this explosion. The following highlights some of the ways in which the media contributed to misunderstandings, which in turn exacerbated an already tense situation. In the following analytical account the reader will find substantial repetition of material already presented in the chronological account. It seemed preferable to do this rather than tax the reader's memory or require constant flipping of pages for reminders.

The Announcement. The announcement of David Levine's appointment in the May 1 *Citizen* was a public relations nightmare. The headline boldly stated "PQ's envoy to head hospital," even though the appointment still had to be approved by the hospital board, which was meeting that same day. About twenty-five board members had been told in late April of three candidates who appeared on a short list, and according to board member Peter Clark there was no doubt about Levine being the clear choice. But at least some members of the board—three or four, by Clark's count—were incensed to find on May 1 that they were in effect being asked to rubber-stamp a decision not only made by the selection committee, but also announced to the media. It was not meant to turn out like that. How did this come about?

Both Maria Bohuslawsky, the *Citizen* reporter who wrote the story, and Brad Mann, who was handling public relations first for the Transition Steering Committee and then for the Ottawa Hospital board, agree on the following details. Bohuslawsky managed to discover the four names of people shortlisted for the job long in advance of May 1. Mann says he was told around the second week in March that the *Citizen* reporter had the information. With a view to sparing indignities to those short-listed people who would not be hired, Mann says he asked Bohuslawsky to hold off on the story and promised to give her more of the story as well as the first exclusive interview with the successful candidate.[6] She agreed to hold off, but her understanding was that she would be given additional information a day in advance of the rest of the media. Mann left Ottawa in the second week of April. When he came back he found that a subgroup of the steering committee had come up with the preferred candidate's name. Mann knew by April 27 that the decision for Levine was unanimous and that the plan was to present the board with the one choice for approval.

Remembering his agreement with Bohuslawsky, Mann phoned her on April

27, thanking her for holding off on the story and saying that he would try to arrange an interview with the new appointee. In talking with her he knew that she had an idea who the successful candidate was. By Wednesday April 29 she knew it was David Levine. Knowing the PR disaster that would occur if the story were published before the appointment was approved, Mann phoned the *Citizen's* chief news editor, Scott Anderson, to explain that the story might turn out to be about the *almost* newly chosen CEO rather than the new CEO if the *Citizen* jumped the gun, because the board might rebel against becoming a rubber stamp. But from Bohuslawsky's point of view, the whole basis of the agreement would be undermined if she were not able to get the story out before the rest of the media. An exclusive interview with Levine would hardly compensate for the scoop she passed up in her original agreement with Mann.

On Thursday morning, April 30, Mann thought he had a verbal agreement with Scott Anderson to do a speculative kind of story, followed by an exclusive interview with Levine. But when Mann, who was in Montreal that day phoned his Ottawa office, a message on his voice mail from Scott Anderson said that the *Citizen* was going ahead with the original story. Mann speculates that Bohuslawsky in the meantime had persuaded Anderson that a special interview was not the deal, and that the deal had involved the *Citizen* being able to scoop the other media.

Brad Mann says he should have realized that the story was just too juicy for the paper to hold off publishing any longer and that he had bought as much time as he could. He says he understands Bohuslawsky's reluctance to be scooped by the electronic media, which would have happened if the *Citizen* had waited another day. Scott Anderson says that when he talked with Mann, no mention was made of the deal with Bohuslawsky, so that when he later heard about the Bohuslawsky deal he felt that Mann had not been "up front" and so his earlier commitment was no longer binding. What special value would there be in an interview with Levine when he would be answering questions from the rest of the media on May 1? Anderson also felt that the board's decision had already been made—why else would they have the elaborate press conference at which Levine would be appearing?

Brad Mann's recollection is different. He maintains that he had in fact mentioned to Anderson the deal with Bohuslawsky, but that the nature of the deal may have been interpreted differently between himself on the one hand and Bohuslawsky and Anderson on the other.

The May 1 *Citizen* headline is worth special attention for its capacity to engender mistrust. "PQ's envoy to head hospital" does not make clear that the new hospital head would be an ex-envoy of the PQ upon taking up the job. An almost indelible image is set up of someone who will be taking marching orders from the PQ at the same time as he will be heading the Ottawa Hospital.[7] Also the subtlety in Maria Bohuslawsky's lead paragraph is lost. She states that "a former political candidate for the Parti Québécois" is "poised" to become the president of the new amalgamated hospital. The headline, however, implies that the decision has already been made, something that would surely be found offensive by members of the board called upon to approve the selection.

Rumours and Speculation. The suggestion that David Levine might be coming to Ottawa to further a PQ agenda was fed by various rumours. Recall that on May 15, Lowell Green asked:

> Mr. Levine—Did you work at the Montfort Hospital during the early 1970s, and Mr. Levine, what is your response to claims by co-workers that at that time you were a *rabid* separatist who refused to refer to Canada as anything other than foreign nation? Has your opinion concerning Canada as a nation and its role *changed* since the 1970s?

The response in the Ottawa Hospital bulletin, "Some Questions and Answers," was that "Mr. Levine has never worked at the Montfort Hospital." Levine was also rumoured as failing to stand up for the playing of the Canadian National Anthem at a New York hockey game. The bulletin further comments that:

> Despite rumours to the contrary, Mr. Levine has not attended any professional hockey games in New York and has always stood up for the playing of the Canadian National Anthem. Also some people are saying that Mr. Levine was required to take an Oath of Allegiance to the Government of Quebec before assuming his position as Delegate General for Quebec in New York. This is also untrue. Mr. Levine took no Oath of Allegiance since this was not a requirement of the job.

I asked Lowell Green by fax on July 13 and by telephone what the source was for the statements from alleged co-workers. I received no reply to my question but he is reported to have mentioned on his talk-show program that he had received my fax. A month later he sent me the following letter, presumably in response.

> Dear Professor Marlin:
> I have no idea why you would want a view from me since it is obvious I am one of those middle-aged fools who don't think we should have separatists running our major institutions.
> It's apparant you have already made up your mind on this matter. The authority of the specially "annointed" people like yourself has been challenged by those who don't have your special understanding of the situation.
> It's called class struggle, Professor. You elitists can't understand

it when ordinary people stand up and fight back. Let me just say that my brain is every bit as keen as yours—my intelligence perhaps superior—my knowledge and understanding of human nature and the political situation is certainly your equal. Why do you believe you are equipped with this special understanding?

I'd also like to know how much this project of yours is going to cost us taxpayers.

Sincerely,

Lowell Green

Lack of Media Support for a Question of Principle. Levine could have saved the community and himself a lot of bother had he stated publicly what he appears to have said to Nick Mulder privately—that he is not a "rabid" separatist, that he has no desire to work for separation and that his concern in working for the PQ was not to encourage separation but to "build bridges" to the anglophone community. What he did say publicly was that he would have no political agenda in running the Ottawa Hospital. He also said that he believed in the right of Quebec to separate if it chose to do so, openly and democratically. He balked at making public his thoughts about whether separatism might be preferable to federalism because he believed in a certain principle: that private political beliefs are irrelevant to competency for a civil service job that largely involves questions of technical expertise. Yes, there is a political dimension, but one of ordinary human relations and not one to which the separatist option has any relevance. To have reassured the Ottawa population any more, by dissociating himself from separatist ideology, for example, would have given tacit denial to the question of principle—the principle that this kind of belief is irrelevant to the job.

It can certainly be argued that David Levine is a symbol of separation, a symbol that is immensely repugnant to Ottawans especially. It follows that, as long as he is seen that way, his appointment is offensive to the intensely federalist population. Therefore, if he is to serve the community well, he should say more to allay the fears of the community. This argument has merit, but so does the argument for protecting freedom of opinion. Maybe the judgement that Levine privately favours a separate Quebec is prejudicial. The New York job may have amounted to a rescue operation by a friend (Bernard Landry) in compensation for Levine's rejection from the CEO job at the amalgamated Montreal hospitals. By not answering more fully the question about his private beliefs on separatism versus federalism, Levine was presenting the Ottawa community with an acid test of its tolerance. Those who believe in hiring on the basis of competence to do the job should not allow personal political beliefs to sway the decision. For Levine to reply to questions about these beliefs would amount to conceding the legitimacy of questioning them. It would also set a precedent for questions into people's political party affiliation, religion, and so on, in future. The question "Are you or have you ever been a separatist?" reeks strongly of McCarthyism. The argument favouring freedom of opinion, however, was not fully and sympathetically aired in the media until the build-up of a fierce anti-Levine movement had taken place.

Repetition. One of the best known techniques of propaganda is the use of repetition. A doubtful claim, uttered with conviction and repeated many times with conviction by others easily becomes a received truth. Statements such as that of MPP Garry Guzzo (reported in the *Citizen* May 8) that Levine was likely to fill "the whole administration with separatists" as he "begins to hire his own staff," and that the "entire administration is going to have a political agenda to break up this country" was repeated in one form or another in talk-show programs, letters to the editor[8] and private conversations.

Rumours were repeated many times. Individuals who believed the rumours repeated them on air, one listener told another, and soon what was speculation became treated as established fact. Take for example the claim of W.G. Anderson on May 7 that "David Levine is a hard-core separatist and has been so since the early '70s." This is assumed true. But on May 22 the *Citizen* carried the banner headline "Levine was once a Liberal, too," with the information that Levine switched parties in the '80s, because he was concerned about the PQ's turn to right-wing economic thinking. Had Daniel Leblanc's May 22 reports in the *Citizen* been published two weeks earlier, a lot of misinformation would have been avoided.

Misinformation encouraged a hard line against Levine and, once the hard line was taken, it became very difficult to dislodge the supposed certainties, particularly when anti-Levine forces identified themselves with patriotic duty. If people fought and died to save Canada in the Second World War, to what lengths should people go to save Canada from separatism? George Orwell once wrote:

> In nationalist thought there are facts which are both true and untrue, known and unknown. A known fact may be so unbearable that it is habitually pushed aside and not allowed to enter into logical processes, or on the other hand it may enter into every calculation and yet never be admitted as a fact, even in one's own mind.[9]

When strong nationalist feelings get hooked to factual errors, it can be impossible to correct them.

Letters. The choice, timing and placement of letters can have an important effect on the judgements people make about public opinion. The letter that appears in the first spot, with the headline above it, will likely be viewed as the most significant letter. With few exceptions, letters were heavily anti-Levine and anti-hospital board at the start. Some of these letters used extreme language, calling Levine a "traitor."

Letters that use abusive language are often dismissed as not worth taking seriously. But when they are presented with many other letters that defend the same basic viewpoint with seemingly solid arguments, it creates an impression that they are not so distant from mainstream opinion.

Editorials and columnists. Until and including May 15, all editorials in the *Citizen* and the *Sun* were negative towards Levine. Editorials carry weight with the public because they usually represent more than one individual's off-the-cuff opinion. They are based on newspaper policy, telephone calls to and from knowledgeable people, letters to the editor, and so on. The reading public learns about a newspaper's obvious biases and will discount editorial views generated from those biases, but it otherwise tends to accord a fair amount of credibility to editorials.

When a highly contentious issue is involved, it is helpful to a reader to have more than one point of view. Unfortunately, the *Citizen* and the *Sun* shared the same negative attitude towards Levine. The restraint that comes from being presented with opposing views was absent at the beginning of the Levine affair.

Ottawa Citizen. The *Ottawa Citizen's* first editorial, May 4, views David Levine as a "Dubious choice" because he had a "close affiliation with a group that has a history of mistreating anglophones," which might "aggravate an already difficult situation." Bilingualism and the language issue, with (unstated) fallout on job prospects, is the only concern. Levine by that time had been quoted as saying he would be "very committed to ensuring the francophone community has all the services in their language," but there is no mention in Maria Bohuslawsky's May 1 stories about ensuring the same for anglophones. Levine may have thought it so obvious as not to need mentioning.

The second editorial, "David Levine should resign," in the City section on May 15, once again makes bilingualism the central issue and argues that Levine will be handicapped as far as reassuring the anglophone population that services will be available in their language. The reason given is that "he has affiliated himself with a political organization that has a history of diminishing anglophones' rights." It further argues that overlooking his presumed separatist beliefs on grounds of fairness would be "carrying evenhandedness to an extreme." It takes the parallel of a prominent member of the Alliance for the Preservation of English in Canada seeking to run a hospital in Lac St. Jean to support the claim that "Political sensitivities do matter."

Nowhere does this editorial look at the possible ramifications in Quebec if David Levine were found unacceptable simply because of his beliefs about separatism. Nor does it acknowledge that people can have motives for working for a separatist party other than that of achieving an independent Quebec. Levine himself said in the interview published on May 1 that for well over seventeen years he had "no link to politics, no involvement in politics" and that he had "no intention of doing anything like that at all." He did not make it easy for people to believe him, but the alternative of revealing his political beliefs would give tacit recognition to the legitimacy of treating the job as a political one. This opens the door to a whole different attitude to civil service positions than one based simply on merit. "Are you now, or have you ever been, a separatist," conjures up visions of Senator McCarthy's witch-hunt of communists during the Cold War. It might also give Quebec grounds, based on parity, for eliminating federalists from its own civil service. Some writers say such discrimination already exists,[10] but if you oppose discrimination by separatists in Quebec you ought also to oppose discrimination by federalists in Ontario.

Why was this editorial so narrowly focused? Perhaps the pro-Levine side were not yet convinced that the worst conspiracy theories about him were not true. Hospital Board Chair Nick Mulder said in a letter dated May 9: "I have always been impressed by the tolerance and sense of fairness which characterize this community." That may be so, but people still needed to be assured that a naive board had not welcomed in a separatist Trojan horse—and there were facts about Levine's past that could have given this reassurance. Information sheets like the hospital's "Questions and Answers" issue on June 9 should have been distributed several weeks earlier. As a result of the anti-Levine propaganda the *Citizen* may have misjudged opinion among the general public and discounted the case for reaffirming Levine's appointment.

When the second editorial appeared on May 15, the *Citizen* held an editorial board conference with David Levine. According to the hospital's PR contact, Brad Mann, this had a strong and positive effect on the attitudes of some members of the editorial staff who heard Levine. Certainly there is a big difference between the second and third editorials. In the third editorial, May 19, "Hospital board must heed public," readers learn of many positive characteristics of Levine, including his commitment that unilingual employees will not be not be shut out of jobs. The central argument of this editorial is that Levine lacks the confidence of the public, though it does not scrutinize whether this absence of confidence is justified or not and does not note the *Citizen's* role in raising public doubt. The editorial concludes by re-affirming its view that the board "must recognize that it made a mistake and negotiate a settlement with Mr. Levine" and it "must be prepared to act on the public's advice." Perhaps the editorialists felt that the relevant philosophical issues were sufficiently canvassed by an article printed immediately below by Reuel S. Amdur of Val-des-Monts ("Loyalty tests create climate of fear," subheaded "Ottawa hospital will be damaged by descent into patriotic hysteria..."). Amdur finds the situation reminiscent of events at the University of California at Berkeley in the early 1950s, recounting the damage done to the university by its insistence that professors sign a loyalty oath or be fired. Amdur states his objection well:

> I believe that an employer buys a worker's service, not his soul .... People of all persuasions have a right to be judged on the basis of their qualifications and their performance, not on their beliefs which are unrelated to the job requirements.

Amdur also argues that rescinding Levine's appointment would likely cause a hardening of separatist attitudes in Quebec: "If we are rigid and rejecting, we will only reinforce the narrowness of the separatists." The *Citizen* can be excused from outlining this kind of concern in its editorial, when the column below does the work. But in view of the arguments in this article, it is surprising that the *Citizen* editorial did not do more in the way of rebuttal, particularly concerning the likely effects of Levine's dismissal on Quebec opinion.

The fourth *Citizen* editorial is equally emphatic that David Levine's appointment be terminated. This editorial appeared May 21, two days after the infamous meeting. The *Citizen* obviously wants to dissociate its own opinion from that displayed by the crowd: "But not everyone who wants Mr. Levine to go is hateful, bigoted, or small-minded—or, despite the impression given by some of Tuesday's video clips, anti-Quebec, anti-bilingualism, or anti-French." It appealed to its own poll showing that 52 percent of Ottawans think Levine should go: "Fifty-two per cent of Ottawans are not bigots." In any case, it reaffirmed, that "After three weeks of heated public debate, it is clear that David Levine should not become the chief executive officer of Ottawa's new mega-hospital."

Adding weight to this position was the unusual appearance of a column immediately below, written by *Citizen* publisher Russell Mills. He argued that despite Levine's superb administrative abilities "his history as a separatist candidate disqualifies him for the equally important political component of the job in Ottawa." The rest of the article is devoted to analysing how the board could have made what he viewed as such a bad decision. But the reference to Levine's "history as a separatist candidate" focuses on his decision to run for the PQ back in 1979, without looking into his motives for running or his later "history as a Liberal" or "history as a superb hospital administrator." The argument reminds us of Earl McRae's comment that "perception is everything." That people perceive him as a separatist, however we define that term, is enough to disqualify him. No room for nuance, no suggestion that maybe people should re-examine the premises in their thinking. The combined effect of the editorials would have provided much fuel for anti-Levine sentiment but, by this time, editorial opinion was being offset to some extent by letters and columnists.

There seems to have been a notable change in the attitude of some of the *Citizen's* columnists after the meeting with Levine on May 15. On May 13 Randall Denley was arguing that the hospital board should be publicly accountable. Though he took no stand on whether the hiring of Levine was wise or not, those opposed to Levine would have found added ammunition in his attack on the board. On May 20, however, Denley was arguing strongly in favour of letting Levine get on with the job. He was impressed by Levine the person, as distinct from the symbol. The upshot was that Levine would be running a hospital, not a country, and that although he "may be a separatist ... he's not exactly Jacques Parizeau." Denley also looked at the consequences of firing Levine: "In the end, we'll be diminished by treating Levine no better than the separatists have treated Quebec's anglophones."

In a third column, "Life after the Levine controversy," May 22, Denley calls for a renewal of goodwill in Ottawa, which has "tried to be a model of French-English cooperation." "There are times in the history of a country when honourable citizens will hold opposing points of view. If we are to maintain a civil society, we must be prepared to accommodate those differences," he writes. Denley says that the board was right to get on with the amalgamation rather than simply turfing Levine out and starting over again. Conceding that there are strong arguments on both sides of the dispute, he concludes that if opposition persists "it will be a fight that will scar our community" and that David Levine is not "important enough to justify the damage this dispute is causing."

Columnist Susan Riley at first defended inquiries into David Levine's beliefs regarding separatism in "Hospital president owes us answers," May 11. Her second column on May 22 repudiates this earlier scepticism about Levine and throws her support behind the Ottawa Hospital board's decision to reaffirm the appointment: "What a relief that the board of the Ottawa Hospital has decided not to bow to our worst instincts—mine included—by revoking the job offer to David Levine."

Riley agrees that Levine's political views have nothing to do with his ability to run a hospital, and analysed her earlier negative reaction as an accumulated anger with separatist leaders that was misdirected against David Levine. She thinks that others may share her annoyance at those who dismiss as "fearful, narrow bigotry" what she sees as "valid, if ill-expressed, anxiety about the survival of Canada." She draws attention to how in the border city of Ottawa "Quebec sovereignty isn't an abstract concept ... or an academic exercise, but a recurring and constant worry." Riley retracts her earlier comparison between David Levine and Jean-Louis Roux, who recently resigned as Quebec lieutenant-governor for having carried a Nazi armband in a rally fifty-five years ago. "There is no comparison and I was wrong and thoughtless to suggest otherwise: The PQ is a legitimate political party—supported by many ordinary Quebecers who are not hard sovereigntists—the other a violent, racist organization."

Riley changed her mind, first, because rescinding the appointment "would be a betrayal of the Canadian values, including tolerance, that we say we cherish," and second, because capitulation to the "braying of a vocal minority and the unease of more moderate opponents ... would have done more damage to this community, to all of us, than to anyone else." To give in, she writes, would have sanctioned meddling by politicians, from Garry Guzzo to Mike Harris, in administrative matters. It would have been used to justify other arbitrary decisions, here, and in Quebec, in which job candidates are judged by backgrounds and beliefs, not their ability. Separatism is a volatile issue right now; next year, it could be some other minority.

Columnist Janice Kennedy also dissociates herself from the behaviour of the May 19 crowd, calling it "nothing less than a national disgrace, a public airing of every narrow, intolerant, ugly impulse that ever peeked out from under a rock—of everything that Canadian mythology likes to pride itself on *not* being" ("Fear and loathing, and a disappointing tale of two cities," May 21). Earlier, she was strongly opposed to the Levine hiring but now expresses her revulsion at being aligned with a "mob of howling bigots that vents its spleen against my native province and against fellow Canadians, inside Quebec and out, who speak French." Kennedy notes as another side of a bad week for Canada, the actions of convicted FLQ terrorist Raymond Villeneuve, who distributed a two-page letter to Westmount residents reminding them of FLQ bombings in the 1960s and suggesting that similar things might be in store for them if they should seek partition from a separate Quebec.

Elizabeth Payne, a member of the *Citizen's* editorial board who attended the May 19 meeting, argues that not only is it possible to show tolerance toward separatists, it is the "only away to avoid public displays such as Tuesday's meeting from devolving into violence" ("Contorting the face of federalism," May 22). In her view it is critical to "break down the wall of fear between Quebec and the rest of the country" if we want to avoid more mob scenes, and worse.

John Robson, *Citizen* deputy editorial pages editor, continued to defend calls for Levine's resignation ("Why David Levine has to go"). His argument? "The sole count of the indictment is that the head of an institution that wants to be a member of a community may not hold views deeply offensive to that community. Like separatism." Robson did not argue that David Levine would use his position to further separatist objectives. Instead he analogized: Suppose Levine had been a Nazi? Would his political beliefs have been regarded as irrelevant? In Robson's view, some political ideas are acceptable and others are not:

> In Quebec, federalism and sovereignty are just two political options. On this side of the Ottawa River it doesn't work that way. Over here, Liberal, Conservative, Reform and NDP are political options. Separatists want to destroy our home and native land. That's why, although separatism is clearly not Nazism, it's equally clearly on the wrong side of the line dividing opinions that don't outrage the community from ones that do.

Robson is expressing an opinion that was fairly widely-held at the meeting of May 19, judging from the applause that greeted like-minded objections. But it is tendentious at the least to state that Quebec separatism is not, on this side of the Ottawa River, a legitimate political option. Many believe that it is a wrong choice, but they understand how some French Canadians might think otherwise. To consider separatism as beyond the pale in Ontario is to lump all Ontarians into opposing a view held by many reasonable, intelligent Quebecers. Robson is entitled to disagree with separation, but he is not entitled to assume that all or even a majority of Ontarians are equally intolerant.

Robson's approach to separatism, like that of many speakers at the May 19 meeting, is governed by a particular threat—the breakup of Canada. Not all who support the separatist party, however, think in terms of a breakup. Other possibilities include a negotiated political arrangement that would give Quebecers more of a sense of sovereignty in their own affairs without necessarily cutting important ties with the rest of Canada. Policies of this kind have been evolving for decades. Some would like that process to reverse, and maybe they are right. Maybe they have good reasons for supposing that the time has arrived for more reciprocity on Quebec's side. But to suddenly label as traitors those who prefer to continue the process is to court an end to civilized dialogue and trigger a downward spiral of hatred and disrespect. The result is depressing to think about.

Robson's column also makes the simplistic judgement that a person who was once a separatist, and who won't say he isn't one now, must be one. That's a bad inference. Perhaps Levine has other reasons for refusing to say more than he did: Quebec has a right to democratically determine its future; the relevance of private political beliefs to the job is debatable; should he be required to work again in Quebec, such a disavowal might count against Levine—why burn bridges when the goal is to build them?

Bill Shannon, an Ottawa writer, contributed a May 28 column that describes how a lot of frustration found a convenient target in David Levine and the board:

> Hiring a man who worked for a separatist government, who was hired in part because he was fluent in French, by a board which was comprised of some of the people perceived to be the cause of job loss, combined all the issues that have been smouldering in the frustration of many middle-aged Ottawa citizens for years.

Shannon thought the affair serves notice to Quebec that all would not be sweetness and light if separation took place: "The David Levine affair is a taste of anger. The PQ spends a good deal of effort trying to convince Québécois and Americans that a breakup will be amicable. The rest of Canada knows it wouldn't."

Shannon is right to draw attention to the feelings of at least a significant part of the population. It is important for the separatist-inclined in Quebec to take stock of the likely consequences of separation. But, on the flip side of this argument, if the May 19 crowd was truly representative of anglophone Canada, would francophones really feel welcome here, given that nearly 50 percent voted for the "Oui" option in the referendum? They might feel all the more inclined to take the separatist option. It's a matter of pride not to be intimidated by hints of trouble to come. Quebec francophones will be looking for the anglophones of Ontario to show a more reasonable understanding of their aspirations and to be a restraining influence on those who shout down defenders of Levine or the board, using hostile words like "treason." The anglophone minority in Quebec likewise looks to the francophones there to show a restraining influence on Raymond Villeneuve's tactics of intimidation. I agree with Shannon that exposure to people's feelings is good, as long as hostile feelings are kept in check.

On the same day and page, Bob Phillips's column on "Quebec's unpaid health tab" draws on the work of Dr. Charles Shaver to criticize the federal government for not forcing Quebec to obey the Canada Health Act. "For about 40 percent of its patients, Quebec pays only $450 of the $745 daily bill an Ottawa hospital typically renders outside its province. This imposes a severe financial burden on the hospital," Phillips writes. The board should have enquired whether

> Mr. Levine's political background is more likely to help him persuade his former colleagues in Quebec to obey the law, or whether it would make him a particularly willing accomplice of the Quebec government in the continuing punishment of Ontario taxpayers ....

This question suggests that Levine should have been hired for his political influence rather than his expertise at running hospitals. We have replied that policy issues of this kind are negotiated at two levels: first, the federal government, to ensure compliance with the terms of the Canada Health Act; and second, the provincial health ministries. Any remaining policy decisions would be up to the hospital board, not the CEO. Ontario taxpayers should also not forget they save money when Ontario patients are treated in Quebec at the lower Quebec rates, as happened in the case of Alan Robinson, who spoke at the May 19 meeting about the excellent care he received for more than a year, two months in a coma, at the St.-Luc Hospital in Montreal. He supported Levine and the dedication to professionalism rather than politics in the health care setting.

***Ottawa Sun*:** The *Ottawa Sun's* editorials are unrelentingly anti-Levine both before and after the May 19 meeting. Only when it became apparent that the hospital board would not back down, after its announcement on May 21, did the campaign to unseat him let up. The first editorial, "Baggage" (May 4), notes that this "region despises separatism and everything for which it stands." David Levine is advised that if he is not a separatist, "he should simply say so," but that "If he is, he should pack his valise and get lost."

A second editorial, "Wrong" (May 16), followed on the heels of the previous day's press conference in which David Levine avoided stating his current feelings about separatism. Levine was "dead wrong," editorialized the *Sun,* "when he insisted his political convictions were basically nobody's business." Because he didn't reject separatism and affirm his belief in Canada, and because he didn't resign, "the new hospital has been thrown into an unnecessary maelstrom, forced to weather the loss of potentially millions of dollars in fundraising revenues in the process." The editorial concludes that the trustees must now "face up to their mistake and terminate Levine's appointment."

The third editorial, "Listen," appeared on the day of the May 19 meeting, noting how the hiring has "deeply divided this region" and urging the board to listen to the public. It also reports that the board itself was divided because only one name has been presented for approval. Said the *Sun,* the board "must revisit the hiring and rescind it—even if it means the hospital will be on the hook for hundreds of thousands of dollars in penalties."

The fourth editorial, "Consequences" (May 22), furious because of the board's decision to stand fast with the hiring of Levine, predicted that "this issue won't simply disappear. It will linger like a festering wound for months, possibly years, undermining public support for an important community institution." The editorial denies charges of McCarthyism, saying that more than half of the people in this region are not bigots. It allowed that some anti-Levine people might "spout anti-francophone or anti-Quebec nonsense. Bright lights always attract a few bugs," but that for the most part the opponents are "sensible, proud Canadians who know the difference between normal partisan politics and a secessionist campaign to destroy the country."

This editorial hints that David Levine might continue to act in the interests of a separate Quebec even while holding an Ontario job and that a kind of blight has been allowed to cross the provincial border: "And they [the sensible opponents] know the difference between a person's right to hold private personal convictions and a person's right to hold public political allegiance. The difference is one of accountability." In other words, Levine may be seeking ways to further the interests of the PQ rather than those of his new job.

This is a prejudicial inference, partly based on Levine's unwillingness to dissociate himself from his separatist connections. But is this prejudicial inference condonable? That Levine would not put political interests above professional concerns should be assumed, since doing so is grounds for dismissal. Forcing him to state publicly that he will not do something so disreputable is demeaning. If he were really so lacking in integrity, he could easily lie. That he chose to remain silent suggests integrity and dignity on his part. Such demeaning requests are characteristic of McCarthyist witch-hunts. As Reuel S. Amdur argued in a *Citizen* article, the end result of this was to demand that people take loyalty oaths, with resultant suspicion and a climate of fear.[11]

The tone of the *Sun's* editorials changed markedly once David Levine started his job on June 15. The June 17 *Sun* editorial, "Welcome Wagon," attacks some demonstrators for their uncivil opposition to Levine:

> A few demonstrators were little more than rabble rousers whose noisy, anti-francophone insults are doing far more harm to the national unity cause than any separatists could ever do as hospital president. National unity is not advanced one bit when francophones are branded as traitorous separatists.

In the *Sun's* view, such people, though small in number, are "having an enormous impact ... in distorting the real and more credible opposition to Levine's appointment." It concludes that there is "very little point fighting for national unity ... if the only way to do so is to destroy it."

Finally, the July 3 editorial, "Heal," approved of some of the decisions made by Levine and the board, noting that they were "clearly trying to be sensitive to the effect such appointments and policies can have on the community."

Columnist Earl McRae deserves to be singled out as the most relentless, impassioned, inflammatory writer, not only of the *Sun* but of any print media. His only rival was CFRA Radio personality Lowell Green. From his very first column on May 14, McRae's language has been rude, taunting and jeering. He opens with a reference to the "thundering stupidity" both of Levine's hiring and his refusal to resign. Levine's political sensitivities are "worse than bush league," and the board of trustees "couldn't manage a one-car funeral." He concludes, "if you won't pack him in, Nick Mulder and Gang of Fools, you can damn well pack yourselves in." This same language was used by Nicholas Patterson, the first speaker at the May 19 meeting. In reference to the May 15 press conference, which was allegedly conducted without translation facilities, he told the board of trustees, "No one but a fool would allow a press conference over 50 percent in French in a country where only 7 percent of anglophones can speak the French language."

McRae's second column, "Let hospital board know you care" (May 18), establishes a mob mentality in a situation that really needed dialogue and critical debate. In a mob setting, only simple ideas carry weight, and heated discussions crowd out self-criticism and doubt. McRae puts everything in simple terms. He speaks of "an incandescent, higher principle" that "marches behind the banner: *Separatist Betrayal, No! Canadian Patriotism, Yes!*" If the board does not admit its "mistake," suggests McRae, it will be putting "ego and cowardice ahead of the hospital and community:"

Tomorrow, Parkdale Clinic of the Civic Hospital, between 6 and 9 p.m. Your chance to thunder. To tell this board to fire Levine or else.

The board will try to turn you around. Don't be intimidated. Don't back off. Don't succumb to doubt. *You* are the boss. Not the board.

Your position is the right one. Shout it out loud.

If you don't show up, if you don't hit the board hard with your red and white heart, if you don't know that you mean business to ensure it can't win, then it *has* won, and you've lost.

Parking in the area is bad; get there early.

For once. Fight. For Canada.

If that's not incitement, it's hard to say what is. There are arguments to counter each of the presuppositions supporting McRae's conclusion, not the least of which is that such raucous fear-mongering by McRae and the crowd sends a damaging message to the French people of Quebec, close to half of whom voted "Yes" in the 1995 referendum and who no doubt resent being called "traitors" when they are seeking to promote the legitimate aspirations of their own population.

McRae's follow-up column of May 20, "Patriots answer call to arms," is full of praise for a mob that was "overwhelmingly united" in their mission to "fight the evil symbol of destruction of the Canada they know, the Canada they love, *their* Canada." That symbol is "separatism," the "Quebec separatism embodied by David Levine; the Quebec separatism embodied by the Ottawa Hospital board of sympathizers that hired the delegate general of the Quebec separatist government office in New York to run the new hospital." These people were responding to a call to arms. The crowd "sang *O Canada* over and over in deafening voice, and they chanted over and over: 'Mulder Must Go!' and 'Get Rid of Levine!' and 'Resign! Resign! Resign!' These were the long, muted sounds of Canada first, Canada only."

Others interpret the scene differently as a disrespectful, rancorous, intolerant undifferentiating mob whose thinking was dominated by imagery: on the one side, Canada and everything good: security, comfort, valour, friendship, harmony; and on the other side, everything bad: separatism, discord, David Levine, the hospital board. There was no room, among the chanters and hecklers, for serious challenges to that dominant imagery. The idea that one of the good things associated with Canada is freedom of speech, and that in their actions they were destroying it, seemed to carry no weight with the loud mouths, nor does Earl McRae see fit to criticize the booing and jeering.

McRae notes that one of the people drowned out by jeers, social worker Reuel Amdur, stated "As Samuel Johnson said—patriotism is the last refuge of the scoundrel." To which McRae replies:

He did not invoke Adlai Stevenson's: "What do we mean by patriotism in the context of our times? A patriotism that puts the country ahead of self ... there are words that are easy to utter, but this is a mighty assignment. For it is often easier to fight for principles than to live up to them."

As mentioned in an earlier chapter, McRae heard wrong; Amdur did not quote Johnson but rather Ambrose Bierce who said that "Patriotism is the *first* resort of a scoundrel." Amdur's point, not surprisingly unreported in the media and unnoticed by McRae in his column, was that:

> The campaign against [Levine] has been led by a local MPP who has shown himself to be a resurrected Senator McCarthy without the charisma, and by two local newspapers noted for their sleaze. Having manufactured hysteria in this case they now demand that the voice of the people be heard, but all they really want is an echo of their own caterwauling.

Amdur began his conclusion with "If Levine goes, it will be necessary ...," but his words were drowned out by the noise of people unwilling to hear what he had to say.

The "mighty assignment" to which McRae refers in his quotation from Adlai Stevenson is that of firing Levine to save Canada, for he concludes his column with the question: "The Ottawa Hospital board hasn't fought for the principles of patriotism; will it now live up to them?" This simplistic reasoning is mind-boggling, even for a populist newspaper without pretensions to being what people normally view as a "serious" newspaper.

Not content with his successful demagoguery inciting the May 19 performance, McRae's May 21 column escalates matters. "Keep the heat on," he advises.

> You stunned, shocked, and shook them to their roots Tuesday night; don't let them think for one second there won't be an uproar they haven't yet seen the likes of if they dare to try to spit in the face of your pro-federalist, anti-separatist Canadianism by winkling in Levine. This is in the best interests of the community? Let them know that if it's civil disobedience they want, civil disobedience they'll get, because there are times and circumstances in the affairs of a nation when civil disobedience is proper and honorable for a great cause .... Keep on fighting.

McRae seems not to know or care about how his remarks will be seen, interpreted and used in Quebec to promote the very cause he is attacking.

Once the board members stood firm, McRae's immediate reaction was to ridicule their stance without suggesting in his May 22 column ("'Howling mob' disgusts board") what action his readers might take. On May 23, he continues the ridicule, mocking Levine's exceptional credentials ("Say a prayer for Levine's health") and suggesting that if Levine is so superior the community cannot afford to let him die. He also argues, as had other commentators, in favour of having the hospital board elected rather than appointed.

On May 25, McRae had still not given up on the possibility of overturning the board's decision. He seems to have had encouraging feedback in the interim.

> I have had more phone calls on this than on any column I've written. All anti-board and Levine. From doctors, nurses, educators, lawyers, francophone and anglophone, professionals, blue collar, all concerned Canadian federalists. These people are not—as the soft-bellied community appeasers are screeching—dumb, redneck, braying morons.

To help his readership continue the struggle, he provides them with a list of phone and fax numbers for each member of the board ("Dial 'F' for freedom of speech").

By May 27, McRae appeared to have found something positive to say about Levine's policy statements ("Common sense not so common"). Most of his column rails against threats to the employment of unilingual anglophones and what he thinks would be excessive bilingualism in the hospital system. The column signifies that bilingualism and the French language are very much behind the anti-Levine sentiment, even though some Levine opponents specify that they are anti-separatist, not anti-French or anti-bilingualism or anything else.

A later McRae column urges continuation of the struggle, not against Levine this time, but against the board that hired him. He encourages continuation of boycotts, cancellation of hospital donations and phoning and faxing board members. The goal should now be a provincial law requiring the election of hospital board members, he writes in "Keep on fighting hospital board" (June 8). McRae draws attention to a petition organized by Ottawa lawyer and editor Carlisle Hanson, Q.C., calling for local elections.[12] This analysis of the underlying problems and insecurity as well as the impact of the media reaction to David Levine's appointment allows us to draw some conclusions about the Levine affair.

Notes

1.   See, for example, the letter entitled "Nurse shocked by poor service at Civic Hospital," *Ottawa Citizen,* May 11, 1998, F5; or the letter from Pamela Watt, Chair, R.N. Council, The Hospital for Sick Children, Toronto, "Why doesn't brass recognize nurses' concerns?" *Toronto Star,* July 29, 1998.

2. Nick Mulder, interview June 26, 1998.

3. Iona Skuce, letter July 20, 1998, and telephone interview July 23, 1998.

4. Regional Municipality of Ottawa-Carleton, "Employee Code of Conduct," (no date), p. 26.

5. As I write this, yet another reason for mistrusting Ontario government assurances appears in the media. In February 1997, the Ontario government announced a $20-million scholarship program to reward excellence. The announcement was made to counter disappointment in and soften the blow of increased tuition fees at universities and colleges. When a student, who worked hard to qualify, applied, she was told the scholarship program had quietly been dropped. See "Ontario yanks funding for promised scholarships," by John Ibbitson, *Ottawa Citizen*, July 22, 1998, A5.

6. According to Peter Johansen, an associate professor of journalism at Carleton University's School of Journalism and Communication, there is nothing unusual about public relations officers making deals with journalists—offering special access to key people, additional information or the like, in return for holding off publication of stories at an inconvenient time. (Peter Johansen, interview July 22, 1998.)

7. It's difficult to see how any headline could have been squeezed into the same space and yet highlight the significant information without being misleading. This case may be an argument for laying out sensitive stories in a way that allows more words in the headline.

8. See T. Conners in the *Sun,* May 15.

9. George Orwell, "Notes on Nationalism," in *Collected Essays* (London: Mercury Books 1961, 275).

10. For example, Lysiane Gagnon writes in *La Presse* (May 23) that it's all very well to defend David Levine's rights to his opinions, but how many upper echelon Quebec civil servants were given cold "thank-you's" by ex-Premier Jacques Parizeau. Norman Riddel was a deputy minister of immigration, but when the PQ came to power they suddenly no longer knew where to place him. Finally he left Quebec. Other people mentioned by Gagnon as encountering trouble for their reservations about separatism were Robert Charlebois, René-Daniel Dubois and Claude Garcia, who was taken off the board of governors of the Université du Québec à Montréal for campaigning for the "No" side.

11. "Loyalty tests create climate of fear," by Reuel S. Amdur, *Ottawa Citizen,* May 19, 1998.

12. This goal has been advocated by many others, including Regional Councillor Alex Munter, who argued against the existence of unelected hospital boards and for health care decision-making by a body directly answerable to the community ("Why hospital boards should go," May 20, C4).

Conclusion

The David Levine affair lasted about one month. Many fears and resentments concerning jobs, language, a sense of justice, and the future of Canada were smoldering in the minds of many residents of Ottawa-Carleton, and they needed little encouragement to burst into flame. The way that the *Ottawa Citizen* announced Levine's appointment "PQ's envoy to head hospital" put front-page focus on elements that would provoke controversy.

Fanning of the emotional flames was sustained through letters, columns, stories and editorials in both the *Ottawa Citizen* and the *Ottawa Sun*, and through rumours discussed on Lowell Green's CFRA phone-in program. It was not until the latter half of May that the weight of material in the *Citizen* tended to counteract anti-Levine and anti-board feeling. Perhaps Levine's meeting with the editorial board on May 15 had some effect. But by that time the *Ottawa Sun* was leading the pack in inciting such feeling.

The media did not invent the generalized fear and resentment, but they did exacerbate these emotions and establish their flimsy connection to Levine. Fair-minded stories, such as the one written by Daniel Leblanc in the May 22 *Citizen*, would have done a lot to drum up support for the board's decision to retain Levine. Why did they not appear earlier? Was it perhaps that the newspaper had decided that Levine should resign?

The *Globe and Mail* provided a counteractive force. Its first report, a well-researched news item by Graham Fraser ("Ottawa angry about new hospital head," May 14, A9), emphasized Levine's credentials.

An important impetus to anti-Levine sentiment came from unchallenged rumours and speculation broadcast on CFRA and published in the *Citizen*—for example, MPP Garry Guzzo's statement in the May 8 *Citizen* that "It's more than Levine now. The entire administration is going to have a political agenda to break up this country." When I asked Guzzo about that statement, he would not stand by it, saying that he was basing his claim only on the general tendencies of people to hire those they know. Perhaps the *Citizen* should have probed Guzzo for evidence of his claims, rather than simply passing them on unquestioned.

A few preliminary lessons can be drawn. The media, in their competitive struggle for circulation and ratings, rely on sensationalism to increase readership and viewership. A majority of the population doesn't care very much for sophisticated analysis. These people like simple stories about winning and losing, where the good side and the bad are clearly labelled. But this formula—well suited to wartime, where the enemies are official and identified—can be a disservice to peaceful co-existence. In political life good and evil are rarely neatly segregated. The demonizing of one side or another serves not to promote harmony but to exacerbate discord.

So, the lesson to the media is simply to show less preoccupation with increasing circulation and ratings and more concern for the general good of society. The lesson to readers is to take note of the demagoguery within the media, or of those who make such a use of the media, and be cautioned against readily dancing to their tune. The lesson for the Ottawa Hospital board, or anyone in an important administrative position, is to be more circumspect in relating to the public. Public relations has become a specialized and complicated business. This means that policies and decisions need PR advice on a continuing basis and not just occasionally and after key decisions have been made. The *Ottawa Citizen's* pre-empting of the David Levine announcement cast a shadow over the actual decision of the board and over the handling of the announcement by other media. It was an acknowledged PR fiasco. Others have suggested that the meetings should have been conducted in a way that would lessen public hostility—by having a much larger auditorium as a venue, for example, rather than resorting to security guards to hold back the crowds seeking entrance to a smaller room. This advice seems sound. Members of the board have admitted to mishandling public relations matters, putting it down to inexperience.

My presupposition in talking about lessons to be drawn is that the May 19 meeting was an ugly manifestation of a hateful side of Ottawa that was all about emotion and very little about reasoned calculation of consequences. Sometimes displays of this kind are cathartic and therefore useful. But they can also be ill-focused and counter-productive. The widely televised meeting was useful to the cause of Quebec separatism but would have been far more damaging to Canadian unity had the crowd succeeded in intimidating the board into rescinding its appointment of Levine.

The hospital board has admitted that it did not anticipate the huge protest that ensued upon the announcement of Levine's appointment. This leaves open a very interesting question: Suppose that the board had correctly gauged the opposition? What then? Would they have rejected Levine to avoid stirring up hostility? How these questions are answered could affect future appointments and will have an impact on Quebec-Ontario relations. The implications affect other matters of tolerance.

More people believed that, once announced, Levine's appointment should not be rescinded than thought it wise to hire Levine in the first place. Reasons included the anticipated cost of a severance package and the difficulty of finding a replacement. Contrariwise, others felt that discrimination against Levine on the basis of political belief would have been all right, provided it was not done officially. These people would not speak of "discrimination," of course, but rather of "avoiding upset to the community."

What does fairness require in this situation? Is it right to stop at recognizing that there will be upset to the community, with the implications for fundraising and the like, or should we further question whether the upset to the community is based on reasonable concerns? My own view is that responsible leadership must go beyond simply giving in to the mood of the public, which can be easily swayed. If the community's opposition is founded on misapprehension, rumours or incomplete information, we should root out the prejudice rather than capitulating to it.

A curious feature of the Levine affair is that, should he prove to be the excellent administrator that his credentials, politics aside, would suggest, then the very arguments made against having an appointed board might backfire. The assumption among many of the vocal opponents of the appointment has been that the decision was a bad one. They support an elected board because such a board would be sensitive to public opinion and would never have made such a decision. But if the decision turns out to have been good, then, if an elected board would not have made it, so much the worse for elected boards. Of course, there are other possibilities, and it is not necessarily a foregone conclusion that an elected board would not have hired Levine. But such a board would likely have at least taken pains to smooth the pathway to acceptability rather than alienating the public by allowing misconceptions to become rooted in the public perception.

It is easy to point the finger at villains, as if all the fault were on one side. The mob arose in anger because deep-seated unease has not been addressed. People value the integrity of Canada and worry about the crisis that would likely be brought about by a referendum won by the sovereignists. They are concerned about the restrictive language laws in Quebec. They sense that arguments for Quebec's right to self-determination and democratic decision-making can conceal a lack of appreciation for the huge burden of problems to be solved in the event of such an outcome. What passes for respect for the principle of self-determination can easily be confused with indifference to the fate of many people whose fortunes would be more directly and more adversely affected than those of the theorists. The flip side of opposition to indifference, however, is the promotion of intolerance, and that would be no less of a disaster for Canada.

If any good can come out of the May 19 meeting in Ottawa, with its display of anger, hatred and contumely, it is the indication that the national unity question can never be set aside. It is tiresome to be constantly negotiating and re-negotiating Quebec's status within confederation, but without an attentive ear to aspirations and grievances on all sides, to the benefits of existing arrangements as well as the ways in which disadvantages still exist and are created, we will spiral into deafness, acrimony and finally violence.

At the time of writing health care has been reliably reported as the number one concern among Canadians. The federal government needs to show its commitment to the Canada Health Act if it is to maintain the confidence of the electorate. The problem of fee payments needs to be addressed. And when a province, notably Quebec, is delinquent, the federal government should either ensure full payment or give convincing reasons why the practice of overlooking incomplete payments is justified.

It would be another positive outcome of the uproar over the Levine appointment, if it encouraged the government planners to do a fuller accounting of the various costs and benefits of hospital restructuring. There are medical problems to be treated, and there are also people. Delivering health services should involve economic efficiency, but not at the cost of infringing on human rights and dignity—either of patients or the health care providers themselves.

For the last two years the policy of the *Ottawa Citizen* under the new editor has been to explore and expose sources of tension in the community, often in a dramatic way. It is debatable whether this policy is the best for the community. It helps to increase circulation, but it may aggravate tensions rather than soothing them. This policy needs to be argued on a case-by-case basis. Whatever the merits of the overall policy, it is still possible to see the good in each case. What the Levine affair has revealed about Ottawa, about Canada, about tolerance and intolerance, and about media influence has been very instructive.

How Canadians as a whole decide to react to this instruction is a different matter. Simply, and obviously, it is up to all of us. I hope that by putting the "Levine affair" under close scrutiny, and by recording, step by step, the development of emotions, prejudices and eventually the display of intolerance, the lessons will not be forgotten. It has been well said that freedom and tolerance live in the hearts and minds of the people. If they aren't there, no laws will preserve them;[1] and if they are there, no laws will be necessary to sustain them.[2] Then again, that's not quite right, because with the best will in the world, people still often need laws for guidance. But the point remains that peaceful coexistence derives from mutual respect and a willingness to listen to those with whom we may disagree profoundly. The Levine affair shows how easily this basic foundation of respect can become derailed. Perhaps it will serve as a useful reminder and act as a deterrent against further intolerance and worse consequences in the future.

NOTES

1. I am paraphrasing Justice Learned Hand, "Liberty lies in the hearts of men and women; when it dies there, no constitution, no law, no court can save it; no constitution, no law, no court can even do much to help it."
2. This thought is partly inspired by the saying of Lord Fletcher of Saltoun: "Give me the making of the people's songs and I care not who writes the laws."

Appendix

COMPAS Studies

COMPAS Studies

The Ottawa polling firm, COMPAS, carried out a public opinion survey about attitudes to the David Levine appointment on May 17, 1998. Commissioned by the *Ottawa Citizen*, the poll results were published May 18, in a front-page, banner headline story. The exact questions are reproduced in what follows. The word "rotate" means that subsequent questions were presented in a different order to different respondents, to neutralize the possible influence of one question on the way the respondent felt towards other questions. With the 410 respondents, the poll had a confidence level of plus or minus five percentage points, 19 times out of 20. The timing of the study was such that it caught public opinion at a time before the backlash against the intolerance displayed at the May 19 meeting.

COMPAS also included questions pertaining to the Levine appointment in a survey August 1, 1998. With only 250 respondents the survey was less reliable, but the reponses suggest that the issue was still alive in August. They also suggest that the Ottawa area population largely favours bilingualism in the Ottawa hospitals. Of course, the question leaves much that is unsaid. No doubt there are many people who think it would be good to have bilingual services in some, but not all hospitals. How would they be expected to answer this question? Many people would prefer a bilingual hospital to one in which only the other official language is spoken, but not to one in which their own language is spoken. So the upshot of the survey is unclear, although a result that says 87% of the people are in favour of bilingual services in Ottawa hospitals gives the impression of a tolerant society. The author wishes to thank COMPAS for permission to reproduce this material.

COMPAS/Ottawa Citizen Survey – May 17, 1998 (n=410)

1. There's been controversy about the appointment of David Levine, a former Parti Quebecois candidate for the National Assembly and former hospital administrator, as a new head of the amalgamated hospital system across Ottawa. Do you think that the newly appointed head [rotate] should be

forced to resign	**52%**
or be allowed to stay on the job	**48%**

* after removal of 13% who don't know or refused to answer

(b) Do you feel that way

very strongly (resign)	**54%**
strongly (resign)	**31%**
or moderately (resign)	**16%**
very strongly (stay)	**25%**
strongly (stay)	**24%**
or moderately (stay)	**51%**

2. How much confidence do you have in the committee that chose him...

a lot	**11%**
some	**33%**
not much	**32%**
or none at all?	**25%**

* after removal of 12% who don't know or refused to answer

3. Please tell me if you agree or disagree with the following reasons that some people say should make him resign. [rotate]

☐ Because a separatist cannot be fair and objective dealing with Quebec, whose government pays less than the full cost of the services that Ottawa hospitals give to Quebec residents

agree	**64%**
disagree	**36%**

* after removal of 11% who don't know or refused to answer

☐ because a separatist is NOT the kind of person to bring English and French together at a time of scarce medical services

agree	**63%**
disagree	**37%**

* after removal of 8% who don't know or refused to answer

☐ because a separatist cannot be successful raising money from either private donors or the Ontario government

agree	**53%**
disagree	**47%**

* after removal of 9% who don't know or refused to answer

COMPAS Research
www.compas.ca

COMPAS/Ottawa Citizen Survey (Excerpts) – August 1, 1998 (n=250)

1. As you may recall, there was concern some weeks ago about the appointment of an official of the separatist PQ government to head up Ottawa's hospitals. Would you say that you are

very concerned	**28%**
somewhat concerned	**27%**
not really concerned	**20%**
or not at all concerned	**25%**
(about the appointment?)	

* after removal of 2% who don't know or refused to answer

2. Turning to a separate issue, would you say that bilingual services in Ottawa hospitals is a

very good idea	**46%**
somewhat good	**41%**
not really	**7%**
or not at all a good idea?	**6%**

* after removal of 1% who don't know or refused to answer

The Ottawa Sun, Monday, May 4

Baggage

The new amalgamated Ottawa Hospital board has unwittingly exposed the real crisis in Ontario's health care system.

And it is this: In all of Ontario, there isn't a single top manager capable of running a major modern hospital.

Yes, from all the available evidence now before us, it appears there was not one single health care administrator from all those closed hospitals across the province that had the right stuff to steer Ottawa's new mega-hospital into the 21st century.

Not one potential president, even from the three merged hospitals — the General, Civic and Riverside — worthy of employment as top gun.

How else to explain the new Ottawa Hospital board's otherwise inexplicable decision to go outside of the province to find its first president, a non-resident Quebecer and former(?) separatist drum beater at that.

The decision is, quite simply, mindboggling — a slap in the face to other candidates who have far more experience with Ontario's hospital system and who have actually paid taxes in this province.

David Levine says he was hired to the new job on the basis of his competency and ability as a health care administrator and that his political beliefs don't enter into it.

We don't question his abilities at all.

But, don't expect everybody to turn a blind eye entirely to his political baggage.

This region despises separatism and everything for which it stands.

Separatists divide Canadians, usually along language lines, they certainly don't unite them.

That's why people want to know whether Levine is still a separatist or whether his past affiliation as a PQ standard bearer was but a brief bout of insanity.

What this region needs in the aftermath of the biggest shakeup in provincial health care in history is someone skilled at uniting people to a common cause.

Someone who can bring together the remnants of three hospitals into one.

Someone who can sooth concerns over language and health services without inflaming one side or the other.

It's not a skill for which separatists are particularly well known.

If Levine is not a separatist, then he should simply say so.

If he is, he should pack his valise and get lost.

David Levine should resign

It's time for David Levine to do the right thing and resign as chief executive officer of the Ottawa Hospital. The public furore over the appointment of the former Parti Québécois candidate and Quebec diplomat has simply created too much public concern for Mr. Levine to be effective in his job.

Donors to the hospital are expressing their disagreement by withdrawing contributions and volunteer time. A prominent physician has publicly wondered whether Mr. Levine will act in the hospital's best interest in fee disputes with the Quebec government. Many ordinary citizens simply believe that a separatist shouldn't get a plum job in the federalist bastion of Ottawa-Carleton. Even Ontario Health Minister Elizabeth Witmer has suggested that the hospital board look seriously at the implications of its decision.

Clearly, Mr. Levine doesn't enjoy the level of public confidence necessary to undertake the complex and delicate task of merging the city's two major hospitals.

The veteran administrator is walking into a volatile situation. The General Hospital has been known as the "French" hospital and now its site will be the dominant one with the most sophisticated services. This has created concern among supporters of the Civic Hospital, who see their institution being reduced to a large community hospital.

As if that weren't enough, the reduced role of the Montfort Hospital means that the merged Ottawa Hospital will be expected to provide bilingual services. For staff, language will be a factor in who keeps their jobs and what kind of work they do. Both French- and English-speaking patients will need to be reassured that service will be available in their language.

It's a difficult challenge and Mr. Levine, despite his years of relevant experience, has a significant handicap in that he has affiliated himself with a political organization that has a history of diminishing anglophones' rights.

It can be argued that it's unfair to deny a Canadian certain jobs because he's a separatist but that would be carrying evenhandedness to an extreme. Political sensitives do matter. For example, a highly-qualified hospital administrator who was also a prominent member of the Alliance for the Preservation of English in Canada would make a poor candidate to run a hospital in Lac St. Jean.

Federalists are offended by the obvious intellectual inconsistency, not to mention self-interest, of separatists who argue to break up the country while wanting to claim all the rights available to Canadians under the Charter of Rights and Freedoms. Separatists demand the rights of Canadians without being willing to undertake the obligations. It's a weak position from which to claim that one is discriminated against.

Those who defend Mr. Levine's appointment say that he's only an administrator, not a politician. Technically that's true but as president and CEO of a major hospital, he's not an anonymous bureaucrat studying files in his office. Mr. Levine would be the hospital's best known face in the community and the person who actually runs the place. He's responsible only to a part-time board of volunteer directors.

Unfortunately for Mr. Levine, his image in this community is not a positive one and that can only hurt his employer, the hospital. It's worth noting that Mr. Levine has made no real effort to dispel community concern or to deny that he's still a separatist. Only today is he finally appearing to answer questions. It's a little late for damage control now. If he says he's not a separatist, will people believe him?

The lack of a timely response from Mr. Levine or any convincing argument from hospital board chairman Nick Mulder has allowed a difficult situation to deteriorate to the point where it's irreversible.

The hospital board has made a mistake and it's time to correct it. Mr. Levine would be doing the best thing for Ottawa-Carleton and the Ottawa Hospital if he gracefully withdrew from the position. Failing that, the board should dismiss him and bear the costs of doing so.

The board says it's responsive to the public. The public has made its views quite clear. It's time to act before this error in judgment becomes more costly.

THE OTTAWA SATURDAY SUN, MAY 16, COMMENT

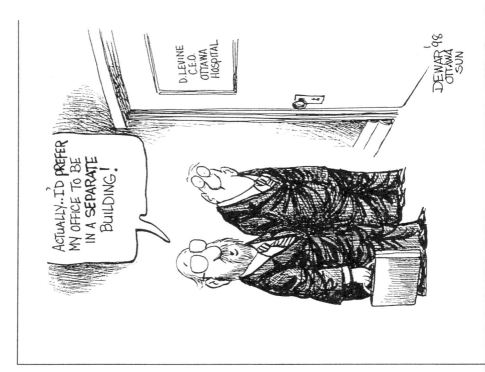

Wrong

We'd hoped that David Levine would have done the right thing yesterday by simply resigning as top administrator of the new amalgamated Ottawa hospital.

Wishful thinking.

Not only did he decline to do the right thing — for himself, the community and, most important, for the new hospital — he refused to do anything to defuse the mounting controversy over his appointment by saying whether he's even still a separatist.

Over and over again he deflected the question, suggesting his political or religious convictions were not an issue.

When it comes to his religious convictions he's absolutely right. We're shocked he even tried to establish a religious linkage to the controversy.

But he was dead wrong, however, when he insisted his political convictions were basically nobody's business.

Well, they were everybody's business when he ran for election for the Parti Quebecois. And presumably they were an issue when he accepted a job as the separatist government's eyes, ears and mouth in New York City.

And they're an issue today, here in a resolutely federalist region, no matter what he thinks to the contrary.

Levine just doesn't seem to understand that residents of this region don't like separatists in their Parliament and don't want them running our hospitals.

As for his democratic rights, he's free to support whatever party he likes. Just don't expect him to be greeted with open arms after publicly aligning himself with a political movement that's bent on destroying Canada and suppressing human rights in the process.

He could have said he believes in Canada. He didn't.

He could've said that separation — especially a destructive movement that deeply divides people along ethnic lines — is dangerous. He didn't. He could have resigned. Again, he didn't.

And because of that, the new hospital has been thrown into an unnecessary maelstrom, forced to weather the loss of potentially millions of dollars in fundraising revenues in the process.

Surely, the board of trustees must now face up to their mistake and terminate Levine's appointment. Their job is to act in the best interests of the hospital and the public it serves.

Better to correct a mistake now than live with its potentially disas-

The Ottawa Citizen, Wednesday, May 21, front page coverage of the May 19 Ottawa Hospital Board meeting

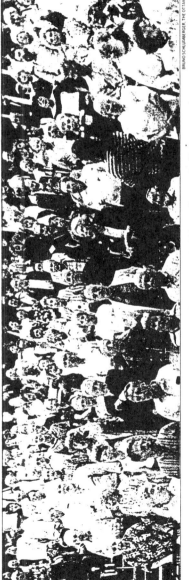

The crowd sings a patriotic O Canada prior to last night's meeting with the board of the Ottawa Hospital. The overflow crowd spilled into a second room.

BRUNO SCHLUMBERGER, THE OTTAWA

The battle over David Levine

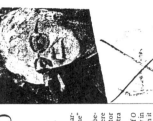

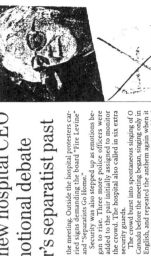

Foes, defenders of new hospital CEO square off in emotional debate over administrator's separatist past

BY PAT BELL, MARK GOLLOM
AND DAWN WALTON

Former Ottawa mayor Marion Dewar and Second World War veteran Daniel O'Dwyer represented the two major emotions last night as close to 500 people gathered to air their views over the appointment of David Levine as head of the newly amalgamated Ottawa Hospital.

"The candidate appears to have fulfilled the requirements for the appointment," Mrs. Dewar said, to a chorus of roars of "out, out, out" from the meeting. Outside the hospital protesters carried signs demanding the board "Fire Levine" and "Separatists Go Home."

Security was also stepped up as emotions began to rise. Three more police officers were added to the pair initially assigned to monitor the crowd. The hospital also called in six extra security guards.

The crowd burst into spontaneous singing of O Canada before the meeting began, singing only in English, and repeated the anthem again when it ended at nine p.m. More than as people had had

Appointed board key to hospital furore

RUSSELL MILLS

How could a group of such bright, capable people make such a bad decision? That seems to be the main question floating around Ottawa this week.

Although we may never know exactly what happened inside the Ottawa Hospital's board room before David Levine was hired as administrator, some speculation is possible.

First, the board appears to have defined the job incorrectly, or at least, incompletely. For the first few years, the job will be as much political as administrative.

Hospital restructuring has rubbed nerves raw in our community. The closing of the Grace and Riverside Hospitals, the national controversy over the Montfort Hospital and the upgrading of the General site and downgrading of the Civic site, a move some are still fighting, have created an extraordinary situation.

The new Ottawa Hospital's top official will have to spend several years making difficult and often unpopular decisions, building broad support for a new structure of health care and healing the rifts in our community.

It's naive to think the public would believe that a board of more than 30 people will make all of these decisions and that the administrator would merely carry them out. The public sees the situation correctly: the large, inexperienced board will be in the hands of an experienced administrator.

The selection of a man with a controversial background for this delicate task was most unwise. While Mr. Levine may be a superb administrator, his history as a separatist candidate disqualifies him for the equally important political component of the job in Ottawa.

Second, although there are many accomplished people on the hospital's board, there are few that have spent much time in the public eye and had significant experience in handling a public controversy. Most are business executives, senior public servants and others who have rarely been exposed directly to the public wrath that politicians deal with every day.

Although it seems extremely naive in retrospect, it is possible to understand how people inexperienced in public debate could think that controversy over Mr. Levine's separatist background would blow over in a day or two.

That doesn't explain how an astute politician like former regional chair Peter Clark could go along with the hiring of Mr. Levine, however. Did he warn them of the possible consequences?

Finally, the structure and accountability of this hospital board are not appropriate for handling a highly contentious issue.

Under our system of government, when important decisions are being made about public facilities and services, the public should be in the room in the form of elected representatives or some other form of direct accountability.

An appointed board may work during normal times when only routine decisions are being taken, but the lack of direct accountability means it is likely to fail, or at least be out of touch with the public mood, when difficult issues must be faced.

When the health minister washes her hands of an appointed hospital board decision, there's simply no direct public accountability at all. The voters and taxpayers are out of the loop.

These reasons, and perhaps others, have led a group of very able people with the community's best interests at heart to make a most unfortunate decision.

The controversy over Mr. Levine has further divided the community and will make it even more difficult to create broad support for a new health care system here.

None of this should be blamed on Mr. Levine. He applied to be an administrator, a role for which he seems highly qualified. It was the board's job to see that running the Ottawa Hospital for the next few years will involve much more than administration. The board owes him a settlement and an apology for hiring him for a job he could not possibly do.

Then the board needs to look at itself and decide whether a group of appointed people with no direct public accountability is the right one to make the tough decisions that will be required to create a new public health care system for our community.

Bad decisions are rarely an accident.

Russell Mills is publisher of the Ottawa Citizen.

THE OTTAWA CITIZEN, THURSDAY, MAY 21, CITY SECTION editorial page

To move forward

After three weeks of heated public debate, it is clear that David Levine should not become the chief executive officer of Ottawa's new mega-hospital.

The continuing controversy over Mr. Levine's hiring has paralysed the Ottawa Hospital Board at a crucial time in its development. Neither the board nor the community can move forward on the large agenda facing it until the former Parti Québécois candidate and current Quebec diplomat has withdrawn from the scene. He could do the community he wishes to serve a large favour by volunteering to go, but if he will not volunteer — and we certainly respect his decision not to — the board should revoke his contract and pay whatever financial penalties seem fair.

After Tuesday's explosive public meeting, it is clear such action should take place as soon as possible. Mr. Levine's hiring has deeply divided the community and it is obvious that, for some time to come, he, not the best way of rearranging Ottawa hospital services, will be at the centre of debate.

Few issues have sparked the kind of anger, hatred and vitriol witnessed in the packed auditorium of the Civic Hospital on Tuesday night. No democrat can condone the tactics demonstrated at the public meeting. Such meetings — indeed, all public meetings — should be conducted civilly. Dissenters, in this case those who support the hospital board, should always be permitted to make their arguments without interruption or, even worse, harassment and intimidation. Such tactics have no place in the Canada that the majority at Tuesday's meeting professes to love so deeply.

Nor, obviously, should the hospital board be swayed by arguments that rely on hatred, bigotry and small-mindedness, qualities revealed in some of the comments and much of the crowd's body language Tuesday night. They, too, have no place in Canada.

But not everyone who wants Mr. Levine to go is hateful, bigoted, or small-minded — or, despite the impression given by some of Tuesday's video clips, anti-Quebec, anti-bilingualism, or anti-French. It is not unreasonable to believe that, in the national capital region, someone who once was a separatist, now is a separatist spokesman, and declines to make clear his views on separatism, cannot win the confidence of the overwhelmingly federalist public whose hospital he wishes to run. The Citizen's weekend poll suggested 52 per cent of Ottawans think Mr. Levine should go. Fifty-two per cent of Ottawans are not bigots. They simply believe that in a country with more than 1,200 hospitals it should be possible to find an excellent hospital administrator who does not carry Mr. Levine's political baggage.

Mr. Levine's departure, like many aspects of his hiring, will be costly to the community. Estimates for adequate compensation run as high as $1 million, a cost for which the 32-member hospital board must bear full responsibility. Add that to approximately $1 million already paid in settlements with the former heads of the General and Civic hospitals and we are at $2 million and counting and still have no one to run the hospital.

In dismissing Mr. Levine, it would not be inappropriate for the board to apologize to him, even at the risk of increasing the settlement to which the courts may judge him to be entitled. He is, by all accounts, a talented administrator. He accepted the $330,000-a-year position as head of the newly amalgamated hospital in good faith. The increasingly ugly furore surrounding his hiring is not his fault.

Fault in this episode lies elsewhere. The hospital board, particularly chairman Nick Mulder, should have anticipated the public firestorm over the hiring of a former and possibly current separatist to head Ottawa-Carleton's biggest hospital. Having taken the trouble to quiz Mr. Levine on his separatist past, the board cannot claim that his political affiliation is of no consequence, as they now apparently wish to do.

Members of the board now have an option. They can admit they made a mistake and get on with the business of helping run the newly amalgamated hospital. Or they can stand by their original decision, in which case they must ask themselves whether they can in good conscience continue on as public trustees, which in effect is what they are.

Mr. Mulder's future is not so clear. As chair, he must bear a large part of the responsibility for the board's costly mistake. It seems unlikely that the board can regain public confidence under his chairmanship.

The Ottawa Citizen, Thursday, May 21, front page

Harris: Levine wrong choice

Hospital board meets to decide CEO's future

BY RICHARD BRENNAN
AND TIM NAUMETZ

TORONTO — The Ottawa Hospital would have been better off hiring a foreigner to head up its newly amalgamated operation than a known separatist, Premier Mike Harris said yesterday.

Mr. Harris is the latest politician to weigh into the red-hot debate on whether David Levine, a former Parti Québécois candidate, should have been named the hospital's new chief executive officer.

"Given that background, and if that's what he still believes in, he wouldn't have been our first choice," the premier said.

"Surely there is administrative capability within Ontario, or least a Canadian or even a non-Canadian who believes in Canada and keeping Canada together," he told a radio talk show on Toronto's CFRB.

The premier's comments came hours before hospital officials met privately to discuss what they would describe only as a "personnel" matter. But trustees have acknowledged that the public outcry over Mr. Levine's hiring has raised the possibility of a reversal.

When asked whether the board would ask Mr. Levine to resign, trustee Maria Barrados said: "We have to look at all the options. Clearly, that's one of the options."

Trustee Pierre de Blois said he is still mulling over the options.

"I think everybody is evaluating the situation," he said.

"(Tuesday night), I think, strengthened my resolve to keep Mr. Levine. It was a totally uncivil meeting, the people opposing Mr. Levine's nomination hardly had any facts — it was a mob. That mentality will probably make me decide to go with the hiring of Mr. Levine because I don't want to give in to that sort of mentality."

The trustees will be meeting all week in private and will issue a statement regarding their discussions, said Judy Brown, a Civic Hospital spokesperson.

See LEVINE on page A2

Levine: Many supporters

Continued from page A1

Liberal Leader Dalton McGuinty said Mr. Harris's comments were "decidedly unhelpful" while trustees are weighing such difficult issues, and added that Mr. Levine is entitled to his own political views as long as they don't adversely affect his job.

"Let's cool down, let's understand what the debate is really all about here. It's quality patient care for the people of Ottawa-Carleton, not the politics of a CEO. Let's not forget our traditions ... that you do draw a distinction between personally held political views and job performance," Mr. McGuinty said.

"I believe it is wrong to discriminate against public servants on the basis of their political views."

Prime Minister Jean Chrétien echoed that view. "In Canada, political considerations are not a question that we ask for employment," Mr. Chrétien said at a news conference in Rome, where he is on a trade mission. "We look at the qualities of the person to serve."

Former premiers Bill Davis, David Peterson and Bob Rae urged Mr. Harris to tone down the rhetoric over Mr. Levine's appointment. The three were in Sudbury yesterday in a rare reunion in aid of a learning centre for people with disabilities.

"I don't discriminate against a man on the basis of his politics, any more than I would on the basis of his colour or religion," Mr. Peterson said.

The ex-premiers compared the Levine protests to flareups such as 1990 the decision by Sault Ste. Marie's council to declare the city English-speaking, and the dispute over building a French-language school in Kingston.

Mr. Rae, NDP premier from 1990 to 1995, quoted what he considered the first rule of governing Ontario: "You never divide the province on language or religion.

"It's essential that you not take sides, but stay in a position where you can be a voice of moderation," he said.

Mr. Harris said he would not directly interfere in the hospital board's decision to give the $330,000-a-year job to Mr. Levine.

"How they spend their money ... is really none of the business of the province of Ontario, but I'm with the people, I would like an explanation as to how this makes sense," he said.

Mr. Harris said most Ontarians would prefer that someone receiving a salary from a hospital paid for by the province's taxpayers should believe in a united Canada.

"I would rather have somebody who is not a separatist," he said. "I can't do anything about it ... on the other hand, residents of Ontario have said they are concerned that taxpayer dollars are funding relatively well-paid positions ... for somebody they believe is not interested in keeping the country together."

Mr. McGuinty said it is a frightening prospect that people be asked their political views before they're given a job. "I think we are beginning to head down a very dangerous path in Ontario when a job interview begins with the question, 'Are you now, or have you ever been, a separatist or a supporter of the separatist movement?'" he said.

Mr. McGuinty, who is the MPP for Ottawa South, said he was troubled by threats that some people might withhold donations to the Ottawa Hospital as a protest Mr. Levine's appointment.

"That wouldn't hurt Mr. Levine and it wouldn't hurt the board members. You know who it would hurt? Our families, our friends and our neighbours who rely on the hospitals for quality health care," the Liberal leader said.

Mr. Levine picked up an unexpected ally yesterday as he tries to defend himself against attacks on his separatist connections. Deborah Grey, deputy parliamentary leader of the Reform party, said nobody should lose their job because of their political viewpoint.

"Nobody should ever be fired for their political beliefs," Ms. Grey said when asked for her views on the Levine affair. "You can do what you want."

Ms. Grey, one of Preston Manning's hardline MPs when it comes to tough action against Quebec separatists, added: "It can go further. It's an unwise path to go down."

Asked to elaborate, Ms. Grey refused, suggesting she suspected she was being led into a statement about the right to hold other political views, such as those advocated by extremist groups such as the racist Heritage Front.

In the Levine case, however, Ms. Grey went on to note that Mr. Levine was a candidate for the Parti Québécois in the 1970s and added there were "all kinds of candidates" in the past who "still do excellent jobs."

Ms. Grey said she was not advising the hospital board or the community. The Alberta MP insisted the decision is neither federal nor provincial.

Bloc Québécois leader Gilles Duceppe called the uproar over Mr. Levine's politics "bad for Canada."

"Is that the kind of democracy people want to live in, in Canada? I don't think so. Any society like that is just showing not a very high degree of tolerance. It's bad for Canada."

With files from John Ibbitson, Dawn Walton, Dave Ebner and Mark Gollom

LeDroit, Friday, May 22

LEDROIT, OTTAWA-HULL, VENDREDI 22 MAI 1998 25

Zola était «Dreyfusard», moi je suis «Levinard»

Voilà 100 ans, presque mois pour mois, l'affaire Dreyfus déchirait la France. En février 1898, quelques mois après avoir lancé son *J'accuse* à la défense de Dreyfus, Émile Zola se trouvait au banc des accusés. On lit dans les descriptions du procès que les commentaires de Zola étaient enterrés par les rugissements inarticulés d'une salle comble. On parlait de l'odeur d'un massacre étouffé, de la haine palpable lorsque se croisaient certains regards, d'une salle de tribunal bondée jusqu'aux fenêtres.

Bref, tout ce qu'on voyait au reportage télévisé de la conférence de l'Hôpital d'Ottawa mardi dernier.

Plusieurs degrés

Comme l'affaire Dreyfus, l'affaire Levine comporte plusieurs degrés.

Premier degré: cette chasse à la sorcière qui n'a rien à envier au maccarthysme des années 1950. Les médias ont beau jeu, ils peuvent jouer les saintes-nitouches tout en moussant le conflit. On n'a qu'à lire l'*Ottawa Sun* pour se rendre compte que, en s'adressant au dénominateur commun le plus bas, on ne vend pas moins de journaux.

Ce qui me trouble, ce que je trouve le plus navrant, c'est cette espèce de bagage anti-francophone qui accompagne toute cette histoire. Je pense au bonhomme qui s'est levé lors d'une précédente conférence de presse, en se plaignant qu'il y avait trop de français. C'est le genre qui, les larmes aux yeux, se demande pourquoi les souverainistes veulent la souveraineté.

Mais quand on ne peut pas s'en prendre aux francophones qui ne sont pas là, il faut «varger» sur ceux qu'on a. La méthode est classique: au nom d'un patriotisme clinquant, retranché dans son infaillibilité, on peut se permettre de mitrailler quiconque ne partage pas nos valeurs, nos opinions, notre parti, notre langue... Comme le disait Samuel Johnson (avec preuve à l'appui mardi soir), «Le patriotisme est l'ultime refuge du gredin.»

Ces gens, ces «patriotes» qui n'enduraient aucun propos autres que les leurs, me font peur. C'est un patriotisme qui pue, qui renie les valeurs de notre patrie. C'est un patriotisme qui sait faire la différence entre «eux» et «nous».

Lorsque le conseil d'administration de l'Hôpital d'Ottawa a arrêté son choix de candidat, il savait qu'un des volets importants de l'emploi était d'assurer des services en français dans une institution présentement anglophone. David Levine a fait ses preuves dans les hôpitaux de Montréal.

Et qui de mieux placé pour accomplir la tâche qu'un vétéran des questions linguistiques du Québec? Un gars de Hipwader, Saskatchewan, peut-être? Il faut s'apercevoir que celui qui vise Levine vise les Franco-Ontariens. Zola était «Dreyfusard», moi je suis «Levinard»

Je suis Franco-Ontarien, fédéraliste convaincu. C'est quétaine, mais j'aime mon pays, je suis «patriote» à ma façon. Mais j'avoue qu'en voyant des spectacles comme ceux de mardi soir, je ne peux m'empêcher de penser: oui, les séparatistes, vous l'avez l'affaire.

**Daniel Chartrand
Vanier (Ontario)**

LeDroit, Friday, May 22, editorial

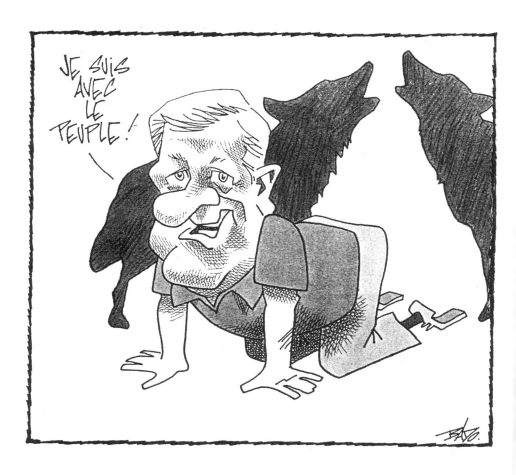

The Ottawa Sun, Tuesday, May 26, front page

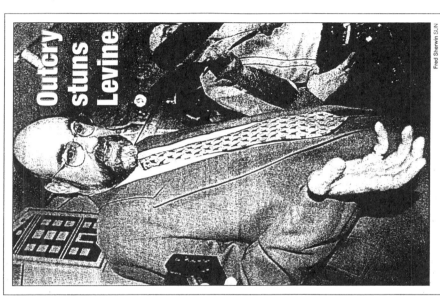

Outcry stuns Levine

DAVID LEVINE gestures at a press conference yesterday to discuss his new job as president and CEO of Ottawa Hospital. The onetime Parti Quebecois candidate said the controversy surrounding his appointment took him by surprise. **PAGES 4-5, 41**

Fred Sherwin SUN

Board axes 500 jobs

Trustees trim $30M okaying $512M school board budget

THE Ottawa-Carleton District School Board chopped 500 jobs from its payroll last night.

Trustees — trimming $30 million while passing a $512-million budget — cut 258 maintenance jobs, 164 central administration positions, 30 teaching and special education assistants, and 41 non-unionized managers.

Most special education programs survived the cuts, at least for this year.

Full story by Donna Casey Page 7

The Ottawa Sun, Tuesday, June 16, front page

Fiery anti-separatist protest greets hospital CEO on first day on job

Raucous start for Levine

CRIES OF "shame" greeted David Levine as he took his seat with the new Ottawa Hospital board last night after his first day on the job.

Anti-separatist protesters gave the new CEO a rough ride, wielding placards calling for the board to resign, and pushing and shoving to gain entry to the meeting.

Only 34 were allowed inside, forcing more than 100 to watch the meeting on a screen in the amphitheatre.

Sol Shinder, filling in for chairman Nick Mulder, was defiant.

"Mr. Levine is not going to resign and this board is not going to resign," he said.

DAVID LEVINE No welcome mat

Story by Sarah Green Page 4

A POLICE officer removes protester Roy Crawford from a scuffle at the Civic site of the Ottawa Hospital yesterday. Crawford was part of a group gathered to protest the choice of David Levine as new CEO of the melded hospital as Levine put in his first day on the job.

Fred Sherwin SUN

Levine protest hits board where it hurts

By KATHLEEN HARRIS
Ottawa Sun

Feisty protesters are boycotting businesses of Ottawa Hospital board trustees who hired former PQ candidate David Levine as CEO.

About 20 demonstrators marched yesterday outside Merivale Mall, where board member Barbara Ramsay owns a Shoppers Drug Mart franchise.

"This board of trustees isn't listening," said demonstrator Tony Silvestro. "Maybe they will if it starts hitting them in the pocketbook."

Carol Dane was also among those carrying Canadian flags and toting placards demanding Levine be fired and the hospital board removed. "They made an error in judgment and they won't correct it," said Dane, a long-time Shoppers customer who is now taking her business elsewhere.

Nicholas Patterson blamed Ramsay and other board members for creating dissension and hatred in the community and damaging financial support for the hospital.

"She has done a terrible harm by supporting this guy," he said.

Patterson plans to continue daily protests outside Ramsay's store, but is also launching campaigns against Peter Burns, who works at Urbandale Corp., and Sol Shinder, who works at District Realty.

A "Sprint Revolution" leaflet campaign will urge people to switch long-distance telephone accounts to Sprint from Bell Canada, Patterson said. Hospital board chairman Nick Mulder works at Stentor, an alliance of communications companies which include Bell.

Ramsay said yesterday she supports peaceful protest, but was "tremendously saddened by the violence" that has erupted in the last few days.

Police were called Thursday when an elderly woman blocked access to the store, verbally abusing customers and threatening people with her cane, said Ramsay. Police are also investigating an incident yesterday when a woman was removed from the store by mall security. The protester called police and said she had been assaulted.

Ramsay said protesters have been harassing employees of her store, labelling her a separatist. She said she has received threatening phone calls and believes she's targeted mainly because her business is accessible.

"I do understand when they see all the changes that they want to voice their concerns," she said.

"But the methodology used is overwhelmingly negative and not helpful."

Ramsay admits the "verbal barrage" could pose a threat to her business, but is determined to keep her volunteer post as hospital trustee. She consulted her 45-member staff and they support her decision to stay, she said.

"I consider it an honor to serve on this board, and until someone tells me I'm not making a positive contribution, I won't step down."

David Green, spokesman for Unity Canada, said the protest was more of a public awareness campaign than a personal attack on Ramsay.

"She and the rest of the board hasn't represented the needs of the people," he said. "We're design. As a businesswoman, she has to be concerned about this."

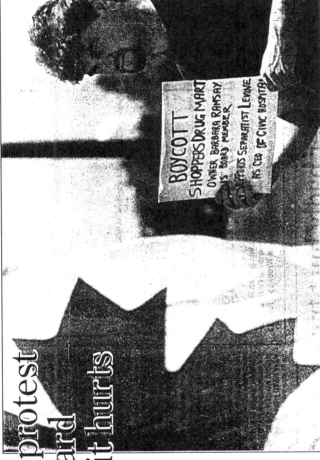

Jeff Bassett SUN

CLIFF PARMETER protests outside Merivale Mall yesterday as part of a boycott of the Shoppers Drug Mart there. Its owner, Barbara Ramsay, sits on the Ottawa Hospital board and backed the hiring of controversial CEO David Levine.

THE OTTAWA SUN, Friday, July 3, COMMENT

Heal

In the heat of battle, he promised to bring peace.

It's been two months now since David Levine, fresh from his job promoting Quebec's separatist government, made that promise.

When the Ottawa Hospital board inexplicably hired him as CEO, keeping him on despite massive protest, Levine pledged to heal the wounds his own appointment had caused.

His first big test, with the eyes of nervous employees and a watchful public upon him, was to appoint a chief of staff this week.

He passed. There couldn't be a more appropriate choice than the man who already holds the job at the Civic hospital site, Dr. Chris Carruthers. A respected orthopedic surgeon, Carruthers has 12 years of administrative experience at the Civic.

And he's a unilingual anglophone.

In normal times, not much would turn on that. But in the tense environment of the General/Civic/Riverside merger, language and politics count almost as much as medical knowledge.

By choosing Carruthers, Levine and the board signal two things: One, that the Civic retains a key role in this new hospital. Two, that bilingualism is not a chief of staff's prime qualification.

(For his part, Carruthers has promised to learn French.)

Levine also eased the fears of many by announcing that unilingual workers will not lose their jobs under the merger. Those jobs, however, can be posted as bilingual when there's an opening — which we fear could lead to more fractious debate.

We trust Levine and the board will apply the same kind of criteria in those cases that they did in Carruthers' appointment — that is, speaking French and English is a desirable, commendable, worthy skill, but it certainly does not outweigh medical qualifications.

After all, the saying "actions speak louder than words" is never truer than in a hospital. What counts is the handiwork of doctors, nurses and staff, not the language they describe it in.

Levine and the board are clearly trying to be sensitive to the effect such appointments and policies can have on the community.

Better late than never. To us, it just shows the power ordinary citizens can wield when they have the courage to speak out.

(But enough with the extremists who insist on labelling Levine "the most hated man in Canada." That's way over the top.)

Carruthers has his work cut out for him. But his appointment puts the hospital in good hands. A surgeon's hands.

It creates a good environment for healing. Fitting, for a hospital.